Dr. Poon's Metabolic Diet

PAT POON

B.Sc. (Highest Honors), M.T. (A.S.C.P., N.C.A.), Ph.D., M.D.,

American Board of Physician Nutrition Specialist

"I can only help those who help themselves."

The information in this book is true and complete to the best of the author's knowledge at the time of publishing. All recommendations are made without guarantee on the part of the author. The author disclaims any liability in connection with the use of this information. The author did not receive any funding from the drug industry in writing this book, and declared no conflict of interest.

People with medical conditions and/or taking medications should consult their physicians before starting any diet or exercise program. Do not alter your diet, or change the type or dosage of your medications without the approval of your medical professionals.

Special thanks to Ms. Maria Wong and Ms. Lis Henry for proof reading the manuscript.

Interior Page Composition & Cover Design: Anie Kim Than

Printed and Bound in Canada
Last digit indicates print number: 12 11 10 9 8
ISBN 978-0-9738905-4-9

CONTENTS

PREFACE

In the animal kingdom, one of the survival skills is the ability to store excess food in the form of fat. The animal can use the stored fat as an energy source when food becomes scarce, for example in the wintertime or in a drought. The human body has maintained this feature even after years of evolution as a means of adaptation for survival. In this day and age though, food is readily available and there is no need for us to store fat.

One way to determine if you are overweight or obese is to compare your weight with your height. This is called Body Mass Index (BMI). The United States National Institutes of Health defines "overweight" as a BMI that is over 25 and "obesity" as a BMI that is over 30. By these criteria, it is estimated that more than 50% of North America's population is overweight. This definition only applies to the North American. It does not apply to the East Asian and Asian. The World Health Organization (WHO) found that, in order to be healthy, the East Asian and Asian populations need to maintain their BMI at less than 23. A BMI of 23 to 27.5 is considered as overweight for the Asian population. A BMI of greater than 27.5 indicates a high risk for obesity related diseases[1]. Recently the Chinese medical community defined "overweight" in the Chinese population as a BMI that is greater than 24.

Is obesity a disease? Due to constraints on health care funding, both the government and industry sources do not regard obesity as a disease so that they do not have to pay for the services. However, you constantly hear in the media and the health care sectors that our population is becoming more obese and people are getting sicker, not healthier. We consider obesity to be a disease when the subject is suffering from conditions that relate to obesity. If the subject is overweight but is healthy otherwise, the subject does not have a disease and does not need to go on a diet. People with hypertension should not eat salt. On the other hand, people who have normal blood pressure and are healthy should be allowed to consume salty foods.

How does one lose the excess body fat and water? Most doctors did not have too many lectures about nutrition in their medical school years. The most common command from a family doctor is to "eat healthy", "eat less", and "exercise more". However, what was supposed to be a "healthy" diet usually made the patient gain weight instead! Doctors later discovered that even with moderate exercise, the patient would still be unable to lose weight if they were eating the wrong foods. There are so many diet programs, books, and dietary supplements out there that patients do not know which one to pick. Physicians should be educated, so that they can give dietary counseling that is meaningful and effective to their patients.

If doctors can help their patients lose weight and eliminate their weight related illnesses, the patients will take fewer sick days, fewer medications, decrease their chance of developing complications, and have fewer hospitalizations. This is a smarter way to use our health care dollars. The government and medical schools should start recognizing obesity as a disease and put more effort into teaching weight reduction strategies in the medical curriculum.

Most commercial diet programs will work for the public, otherwise they would cease to exist. However, as medical practitioners, doctors are dealing with a different type of clientele. Our patients all have medical conditions that relate to obesity. The diet plan for this type of patient will have to be customized to fit their needs. These patients need to be followed more closely than the healthy obese patients. A patient who has Type 2 diabetes, hypertension, high cholesterol and a high triglycerides level will be taking many medications, and during the weight loss process, the type and dosage of medications may need to be modified and their blood chemistry monitored. Many medical conditions and medications can cause patients to weight gain. Simply going to a weight loss clinic and being given a set meal plan, purchasing prepared diet food, or relying on diet pills and vitamin injections may not be in the best interest of this type of obese patients. It can even endanger the patient's health if the diet clinic does not know how to monitor the patient's condition. The patient's family doctor is the ultimate person in charge of the patient's health. Therefore, our clinic insisted that the family doctors should be responsible for referring their patients to us and that the family doctor should be involved in all the major decision processes. We do not accept patients to our program without the approval of their family doctor.

A good diet plan should have a sound biochemical theory behind it. It should be simple, easy to follow and have a low complication rate. The patients should be allowed to eat whenever they feel hungry and see results within a short period of time. Patients should be able to maintain the weight once the goal is reached. The diet program should involve more than just providing the patient with a set menu, it should provide an opportunity to teach the patients and their families about nutrition. The Dr. Poon's Metabolic Diet program goes beyond teaching patients about "healthy eating". For example, following the Canadian Food Guide for Healthy Eating may not be able to help the patients to lose weight or improve their medical conditions.

The first part of this book is written specifically to teach medical professionals about obesity, nutrition and diseases. The second part is less technical, and provides the actual diet plan to the patients. It is less technical. This book provides explanations and scientific evidence disproving common misconceptions about dieting so that the patient can follow this diet without reservation. A list of the sugar and starch contents of common food items can be found in the appendix so that the patient can make better food choices.

Reference:

1. WHO Regional Office for the Western Pacific/International Association for the Study of Obesity/International Obesity Task Force. The Asia-Pacific perspective: redefining obesity and its treatment. Sydney, Health Communications Australia 2000.

1 : OBJECTIVES

* To combat obesity related diseases
* To lose fat and excess water weight
* To preserve muscle and bone
* To lose weight quickly and safely
* To keep weight off for life

We started this diet program a few years ago to help our patients with medical problems secondary to their obesity. After a ten-percent reduction in their weight, most of their medical problems became less severe, if not totally eliminated. This is particularly true for patients with metabolic syndrome, Type 2 diabetes, hypertension, indigestion, gastroesophageal reflux, high serum triglycerides, high serum cholesterol, polycystic ovarian syndrome, fluid retention, sleep apnea, arthritis, and fibromyalgia. Surgical patients were frequently referred to us by their surgeons to help them lose weight pre-operatively to lower their peri-operative and post-operative morbidity and to decrease the chances of disease recurrence.

Metabolism is the set of chemical reactions that occur in living organisms in order to maintain life. These processes allow organisms to grow and reproduce, maintain their structures, and respond to their environments. Metabolism is usually divided into two categories: Catabolism and anabolism (Fig. 1). Catabolism breaks down organic matter for purposes such as harvesting energy in cellular respiration. Anabolism, on the other hand, uses energy to construct components of cells such as proteins and nucleic acids.

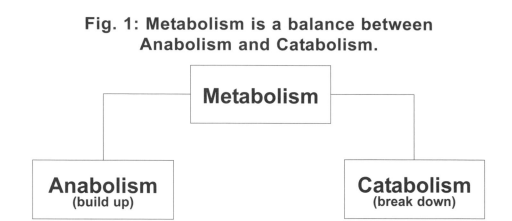

Fig. 1: Metabolism is a balance between Anabolism and Catabolism.

When the anabolic rate is equal to the catabolic rate, the body is in equilibrium, and there will be no change in weight. When the catabolic rate is higher than the anabolic rate, the patient will lose weight. The objective of this diet program is to provide an environment that favors catabolism of fat and anabolism of protein. This diet is designed to help the patient lose body fat, especially the fat that is around the waist area (which is deemed a risk factor for heart disease), and to maintain the lean muscle mass. The net effect will be to lose inches from your waistline and to decrease your percentage of body fat. This book will show you that it is not *how much* you eat but *what* you eat that causes you to gain weight in the first place. None of our patients have ever told us that their reason for gaining fat in the abdomen was that they ate too much fatty meat, but rather from eating too many carbohydrates.

Many patients have told us that they do exercise routinely and *watch* their diets, however, they still end up with weight gain. This is because exercise without the proper diet will not work unless you are doing hours and hours of cardiovascular exercise every day and decrease your daily calorie intake at the same time. The problem with the calorie-counting type of diet is that the patient feels hungry a lot of the time. If a doctor tells the patient not to breathe and the patient tried his best not to breathe, how long would he stop breathing? Not for very long. As a survival instinct, the brain will take charge and force the patient to breathe. The brain will not allow the patient to suffocate regardless of willpower. Eating is the same. The patient can starve for a few days and lose some weight. Eventually the brain will make the patient eat. If the patient consumes the wrong foods, he is going to regain the weight.

This diet will allow patients to eat as much as they need to satisfy their hunger, and they will lose weight at the same time. With the proper diet, the patient will lose more fat and excess water than muscle. With the proper exercise, the patient will regain the lost muscle.

When patients tell us that they are *"watching their diet"*, they usually mean that they are eating less fat and meat because they were told that eating meat is not healthy. Even when our patients tell us that they are following a low-carb diet, after going over their food diary, we often find that their diets are high in carbohydrates. That is because people only consider bread and pasta as carbohydrates and do not know that there are many more food items that are full of hidden carbohydrates. Patients also try to avoid seafood because of the belief that seafood, especially shellfish, is high in fat and cholesterol. This book will show you that you can eat meat, seafood and shellfish, and still improve your lipid profiles.

While you are on this program, your bodily functions will need to be monitored to make sure that you are proceeding with the diet correctly and that your body is not suffering from any adverse complications. You will be required to do blood and urine testing regularly as needed. This diet is completely safe if followed properly. By following this diet plan diligently, you will be burning off fat 24 hours a day, even while you are sleeping! Typically, a patient will lose an average of 7 to 10 pounds during the first two weeks of the *Induction Phase (Phase 1)*. A loss of 1.5 to 3 pounds weekly is common during the *Continued Weight Losing Phase (Phase 2)*. It depends on your initial weight. Most patients can achieve a 10% weight loss every two months on Phase 2. Once you have achieved the necessary weight loss, we will then show you how to eat properly and maintain your weight and health during the *Maintenance Phase (Phase 3)*.

We do not claim that this is a miracle diet, and this diet may not be suitable for everybody. Try this diet for eight weeks and see for yourself how well you will feel and look after a 10% reduction in your weight.

"Seafood dinner - $ 20.00
New pants - $ 65.00
Losing 10% of your weight - Priceless"

2: WHAT IS OBESITY

Recognized since 1985 as a chronic disease, obesity is the second leading cause of preventable death, exceeded only by cigarette smoking. Approximately one-third of adults are estimated to be obese. Approximately one in five children in the United States between the ages of 6 and 17 are overweight. This number is on the rise.

There is a difference between the terms *"overweight"* and *"obesity"*. *"Overweight"* means that there is an excess of total body weight, which includes muscle, fat, bone, water, and blood in relation to height. *"Obesity"*, on the other hand, means that there is an excess of body fat only. Hence, a body builder may be overweight but not obese, because he has a high level of lean body mass. This is why measuring the patient's weight alone does not tell the whole story about the patient's body composition. Measurement of the body fat percentage is also important.

According to the National Institutes of Health, an increase in body weight of 20 percent or more above the desirable weight is the point at which excess weight becomes a health hazard.

A good way to estimate if someone is overweight or obese is by measuring the Body Mass Index (BMI). The Body Mass Index can be calculated using the following formula.

$$\frac{\text{Weight (kg)}}{\text{Height (m)}^2}$$

If your weight is 90 kilograms and your height is 1.62 meters, then your BMI will be 34.

> BMI 20 to 25 = Normal
>
> BMI > 25 = Overweight
>
> BMI > 30 = Class 1 Obesity
>
> BMI > 35 = Class 2 Obesity
>
> BMI > 40 = Morbid Obesity Class 3

When someone is labeled as overweight, that person has to have a body mass index of great than 25 but less than 30. This is true in both men and women. When your BMI is over 30, you are classified as obese. Most studies show an increase in mortality rate associated with obesity. Obese individuals have a 50 to 100 percent increased risk of death from all causes, compared with normal-weight individuals (BMI 20-25). Most of the increased risk is due to cardiovascular causes. Life expectancy of a moderately obese person could be shortened by 2 to 5 years. Caucasian men between 20 to 30 years old with a BMI > 45 could shorten their life expectancy by 13 years; Caucasian females in the same category could lose up to 8 years of life. Young African American males with a BMI > 45 could lose up to 20 years of life; African American females, up to 5 years.

The above BMI classification only applies to the North American population. The Asian (India and Far East) population has a different classification scale. Normal weight Asians should have a BMI of 20 to 23. A BMI over 23 is classified as overweight and a BMI over 27 is classified as obese.

Obesity can also be determined by your height, waist, hip and wrist circumferences, or waist to hip ratio, or using a caliper, or CT scan. When a man has a body fat percentage greater than 20% and a woman has a body fat percentage greater than 32%, he or she is considered to be obese. The normal waist to hip ratio for a male is 1, and for a female is 0.8. Unlike BMI, these normal values are age specific.

Obesity can lead to diabetes, insulin resistance, hyperinsulinemia, hypercholesterolemia, hypertriglyceridemia, low levels of high density lipoprotein (HDL) cholesterol, sleep apnea, heart burn, arthritis, inflammatory bowel disease, polycystic ovary syndrome, hypertension (high blood pressure), gout, gallbladder disease, coronary heart disease, and cancers of the endometrium, ovary, cervix, breast, colon, rectum, kidney, esophagus, gallbladder and prostate. In a study investigating the effects of excess weight on cancer-related deaths, researchers evaluated 900,000 patients for 16 years. They concluded that excess weight might account for 14 percent of all cancer-related deaths in men and 20 percent of those in women.

Obese patients are surgical risks as well. Not only does mortality increase 3-fold among obese patients, but they are also more prone to postoperative complications.

The body fat distribution is also important. Excess fat in the abdominal region (more common in males) is associated with a significant increase in risks for many medical conditions. A waist circumference of greater than 36 inches (91 cm) for females and 40 inches (102 cm) for males is correlated with a higher risk of developing coronary heart disease. However, the numbers only pertain to the North American population, and do not apply to Asians. A new set of numbers has been assigned to the Asian population. The maximum waist circumference for Asian males is 36 inches (91 cm) and 32 inches (81 cm) for Asian females. The latest research showed that for Asian males, the waist circumference should be below 33 inches (84 cm) and for Asian females is 29 inches (74 cm)[1]. Please note that the BMI and waist circumference numbers are for adults only and do not apply to children. The mean waist circumference and the prevalence of abdominal obesity among U.S. adults have increased continuously during the past 15 years[2].

To measure your waist circumference accurately, first locate the top part of your hipbone on the side of your body underneath the armpit. Then, locate the lowest rib right above the hipbone. Take a point halfway between these two marks and wrap the measuring tape around your abdomen. The tape should be parallel to the floor. Take the measurement as you exhale.

Abdominal obesity is associated with high levels of serum insulin, and all the other risks of high insulin. Fat that is in the hip area (more common in female) carries a lower risk of chronic diseases. When you see fat in the waist area, you know that fat is also building up inside the abdominal cavity, around your organs and infiltrating your liver and pancreas.

To determine which weight category you belong to, BMI, body fat percentage (using a scale with impedance measurement capacity) and waist circumference should be measured. If your BMI, body fat percentage and waist circumference are high, you have abdominal obesity (apple-shaped). This will increase your risk of the diseases mentioned above. However, when the BMI is high, and the body fat percentage and waist circumference are normal, you are not as at risk for developing those diseases (pear-shaped).

The measurement of waist circumference does *not* change the treatment approach for those who have a BMI greater than 30, i.e., no matter what the waist circumference is, once you have BMI of over 30, your treatment will be the same[3]. Among normal weight or obese women and men (regardless of BMI category) waist circumference did not appear to substantially add to the predictive value of risk for vascular events[4]. Sometimes it can be unpractical to measure waist circumference in our office when we see a patient for the first time. This is because measurement of the waist circumference is done on bare skin and patients have to remove items of clothing in order to expose the area of interest. Since all of our patients have a BMI of over 30 and we measure body fat percentages on each one, we seldom measure the patient's waist circumference.

It is imperative to recognize that there are many different factors that cause obesity. We will try to identify the reasons behind your obesity and find the right solution accordingly.

The most common reason for developing obesity is due to a high calorie intake (overeating) compared to the amount of energy expended. Which macronutrients cause obesity? Of the three major food groups (protein, fat, and carbohydrate), it is the over-consumption of carbohydrates that causes the most weight gain. The World Health Organization technical report series 916, Geneva 2003 stated that sugar and starch are energy dense and promote weight gain. During the past decade, the amount of fat consumption as a percentage of daily caloric intake has been on a decline. Yet the population is becoming more obese. This is because we are eating more carbohydrates and less protein and fat.

Dietary fat, energy density, sugar and carbohydrates were all implicated in the development of obesity. However, there as no linkage between protein consumption and obesity. Increasing intake of carbohydrates and fats may have contributed to the prevalence of obesity and Type 2 diabetes observed in Canada during the last two decades[5]. In the Nurse Health Study, it was found that the percentage of caloric intake from fat has only a weak positive association with weight gain[6].

Many patients who come to see us regarding their weight problem tell us that there must be something wrong with their metabolism and that their hormones must be abnormal. Yes, hormonal problems can be related to obesity. However, most of these hormone abnormalities will show up early in life and are usually present with mental retardation or developmental delay and hypogonadism. Diseases such as Prader-Willi Syndrome, Bardet-Biedl Syndrome, hypothalamus tumors, prolactinomas, chromosomal abnormality, growth hormone deficiency, and pseudohypoparathyroidism are very uncommon. Patients with any of the above diseases will experience many more signs and symptoms than just weight gain.

Disease of the thyroid (hypothyroidism), adrenal glands (Cushing syndrome), and Polycystic Ovary Syndrome, happen later in life and are not uncommon. Hypothyroidism may be the end result of a number of diseases of the thyroid gland or it may be secondary to pituitary failure and medication. Hypo means low. Hence, patients with hypothyroidism will have a decreased level of thyroid hormone in their blood. The net effect will be a lower basal metabolic rate, leading to cold intolerance and weight gain, coarse and sparse hair, dry and yellowish skin, and a husky voice. Simple blood, urine and radiological examinations can easily help us in making the correct diagnosis.

There are genetic factors that influence eating behavior, but research is still ongoing at this time.

Certain medications can cause weight gain. The mechanism of weight gain varies from simple water retention to induced hunger sensations, to complicated biochemical manipulations (Chapter 10).

Obesity is about excess fat. One has to know a bit about the anatomy and physiology of the fat tissue. What you call fat, the doctor calls *"adipose tissue"*. What you call fat cell, the doctor calls *"adipocytes"*. What you call fat in the blood, the doctor calls "triglycerides". Adipose tissue consists of pre-adipocytes, adipocytes, sympathetic nerves, macrophages and capillaries. Ten percent of the adipocytes content is water, and the rest is mainly fat. The body can store an infinite amount of fat because pre-adipocytes can divide themselves to create extra storage space for fat. It was shown that it is the number of adipocytes that correlates with insulin resistance. Only pre-adipocytes can divide but not the mature adipocytes.

There are a few factors that can increase the rate of fat formation. Activation of peroxisome proliferator-activated receptor gamma (PPAPγ) is essential to adipocytes formation. Activation of this receptor can be accomplished by insulin, adiponectin, fatty acid, glucose and amino acid.

References:

1. Waist Circumference and BMI Cut-off Based on 10-year cardiovascular risk: Evidence for "Central Pre-Obesity". Obesity 2007;15: 2832-39.

2. Li, C., Ford, E.S., McGuire, L.C., et al. Over one-half of U.S. adults had abdominal obesity in the period of 2003-2004. Obesity 2007;15: 216-223.

3. Klein, S, Allison, DB, Heymsfield, SB, et al. Waist circumference and cardiometabolic risk: a consensus statement from shaping America's Health: Association for weight management and obesity prevention; NAASO; and the American Diabetes Association. Obesity. 2007;15:1061-67.

4. Matthew Freiberg, Michael Mencina, Ralph D'Agostino et al. BMI vs. Waist Circumference for identifying vascular risk. Obesity 2008;16:463-69.

5. Mo F., Morrison H., Choi B., Impact of energy intake from carbohydrate, fat and protein related to obesity and Type 2 diabetes in Canada. Canadian Journal of Diabetes. 2006;30:284.

6. Field A, Willett W, Lissner L. Dietary fat and weight gain among women in the Nurse Health Study. Obesity 2007;15:967-76.

"If you don't lose, don't gain."

3: Complications Associated with Obesity

In this chapter, we will discuss some of the co-morbidities that caused by obesity. There are potential signs and symptoms associated with obesity (Table 1).

Table 1. Signs and Symptoms Commonly Found in Obese Patients.	
Appearances	**Symptoms**
Increase in size of waistline, neck size, etc	Shortness of breath
Thinning of hair	Tiredness, loss of energy
Increase in facial and body hairs in women	Somnolence
Water retention such as swollen feet, hands, and ankles	Poor concentration and memory
Thickened skin fold at the back of the neck and armpits	Painful joints and back, gout
Skin tags around the neck and armpits	Heart burn, indigestion, gallstone attack
Acne	Snoring
Gynecomastia - enlargement of the male breast	Sweating
Walking with a wide gait	Deep vein thrombosis
Protrusion of the abdomen	Rapid heart beats
Stretch marks on skin	Light-headedness
Buffalo hump below the back of the neck	Depression, loss of interest
Bow legged or knock knees secondary to arthritis of the knees	Low self-esteem
Shortness of breath	Impotence
Fatty deposits on upper eyelids	Infertility
Varicose veins	Irregular period
Discoloration at the lower limbs	Recurrent skin infection, vaginal infection, cellulitis

Just as a doctor is ever vigilant in patients who are heavy smokers, who may or may not develop lung cancer, doctors must examine their obese patients for the following group of diseases that have the potential to develop. Especially if there is a positive family history of one or more of these diseases:

1. Type 2 diabetes

2. Hypertension, dyslipidemia and coronary heart disease

3. Obesity and cancer

4. Autoimmune disease

5. Acne and other skin disorders

6. Water retention

7. Polycystic ovarian syndrome

8. Liver disease

9. Osteoarthritis

10. Sleep apnea

11. Hyperuricemia

12. Fibromyalgia and chronic fatigue syndrome

Type 2 Diabetes

Type 2 (adult onset) diabetes accounts for nearly 90% of all cases of diabetes (Figure 2). Researchers estimate that over 95% of Type 2 diabetes cases diagnosed in obese people are a direct result of their obesity. Even if the obese patient is not diabetic at the time, an increase in 1 kg (2.2 pounds) per year translates into a 49% increased risk of the developing diabetes within the next 10-years. This is the type of patient that we are interested in treating with our diet plan.

Figure 2. Over Eighty-Five Percent of all Newly Diagnosed Diabetics are Overweight.

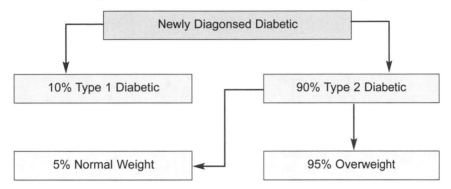

Type 2 diabetics are able to produce insulin on their own. Nevertheless, due to their obesity (especially the abdominally obese type), they have to secrete an even higher amount of insulin than normal patients in order to fight insulin resistance and to handle the sugar load that they ingest daily. However, sometimes the excess amount of insulin produced is still not enough for the overweight body and the doctor has to give the patient medications to help the patient to produce even more insulin. This leads to *Hyperinsulinemia* and causes further weight (fat) gain. As they gain more fat weight, they require more insulin production and thus higher doses of medications will be prescribed. The vicious cycle begins. Worldwide, the number of cases of diabetes is currently estimated to be around 150 million. This number is predicted to double by 2025, with the greatest number of cases being expected in China and India. This may be due to the more affluent lifestyle they will enjoy when their countries become more prosperous. Previously a disease of the middle-aged and elderly, Type 2 diabetes has recently escalated in all age groups and is now being identified in younger and younger age groups. Both patients and doctors alike are more conscious about diabetes and early detection leads to early diagnosis.

The type of diet that promotes diabetes is typically energy-dense, high in saturated fatty acids and depleted in fibers (Table 2).

Table 2. Summary of Strength of Evidence on Lifestyle Factors and Risk of Developing Type 2 Diabetes.

Evidence	Decreased Risk	Increased Risk
Convincing	Voluntary weight loss in overweight and obese people Physical activity	Overweight and obesity Abdominal obesity Physical inactivity Maternal diabetes
Probable	Dietary fiber	Saturated fats Intrauterine growth retardation
Possible	Omega-3 fatty acid Exclusive breastfeeding Low glycemic index foods	Total fat intake Trans fatty acids
Insufficient	Vitamin E Chromium Magnesium Moderate alcohol	Excess alcohol

(Adapted from WHO Technical Report Series 916, 2003.)

The treatment of obese Type 2 diabetes in the early stage should be through diet control and exercise, not by medications. It is the elimination of excess fat that control this type of diabetes. It is the weight that causes the disease in the first place. In fact, putting a patient on certain medications can make the problem worse in some cases.

In the past, fat and protein were seen as the enemies of diabetics, and a high-carbohydrate diet was the mainstream treatment. At one time, the American Diabetes Association recommended a 60 percent carbohydrate diet for the treatment of diabetes. Nowadays, the carbohydrate recommendation is lower.

This diet is low in absorbable carbohydrates (net carbohydrates), which means that your body does not have to secrete an extra amount of insulin to handle the sugar load. Once you decrease your fat weight, your body will no longer need the extra insulin to compensate for insulin resistance, and thus hyperinsulinemia is slowly eliminated. I hope that you will be able to eliminate some of your anti-diabetic medications. If you have to take any medications, it will be for the prevention of a diabetic flare up and/or to preserve the Beta cell function (the pancreatic cells that produce insulin). This is determined by the stage of your Type 2 diabetes. As a general rule, the longer you are diabetic, the more difficult it is to get rid of all your medications. The longer you are diabetic, the more likely it is that you will end up relying on insulin injection. The longer your diabetes is out of control, the more likely that you will suffer from diabetic complications.

Mechanism of Obesity Induced Type 2 Diabetes

In order to design a diet to treat Type 2 diabetes, we need to look into the mechanism by which obesity promotes Type 2 diabetes. We have shown you earlier that it is the ingestion of carbohydrates that causes obesity in the first place. We are going to show you a simplified version of the usual pathway of carbohydrate metabolism in a *healthy non-obese patient*.

The human body has a regulation mechanism that maintains the blood glucose within a narrow range (3.5 to 5.6 mmol/L fasting). After ingestion of a carbohydrate rich meal (e.g. a piece of bread), the blood glucose rises and triggers, the secretion of insulin from the Beta cells of the pancreatic islet. Insulin increases the glucose uptake by muscle and liver cells. Glucose acts as the main source of fuel for energy production. If there is a lot of extra glucose in the blood, insulin will promote the muscle and liver cells to store the glucose as glycogen (glycogenesis). At the same time, insulin suppresses the break down of glycogen (glycogenolysis), decreases the release of fatty acid from fat cells (lipolysis) and inhibits the production of glucose by the liver cells (gluconeogenesis). This will bring the blood glucose level back to normal.

After fasting for more than ten hours, blood glucose levels will go down. Low blood glucose levels will stop the secretion of insulin. Another hormone called *glucagon* will be secreted from the pancreatic

Alpha cells instead. Glucagon promotes the breakdown (oxidation) of muscle and liver glycogen and changes glycogen back into glucose to use as fuel for the bodily functions. Glucagon also promotes gluconeogenesis in the liver, and to a lesser degree, in the muscles. During gluconeogenesis, protein is metabolized and converted into glucose. Under the influence of glucagon, lipolysis occurs in the adipose tissue and part of the fat molecule also turns into glucose. All of these mechanisms will bring the blood glucose level back to normal. When the patient eats, the blood glucose level comes up and triggers insulin secretion and inhibits the secretion of glucagon. The whole process then repeats itself. This is what happens to the blood glucose in a non-obese, non-diabetic patient.

Now, let us say that this patient decides to increase his carbohydrate intake and to stop exercising. The extra glucose in the blood will be stored as glycogen in the liver and muscles, with the help of insulin as mentioned above. However, the patient keeps on eating carbohydrates and the liver and the muscle have no more space to make or to store glycogen. Under the influence of insulin, the extra glucose will now be converted into *fatty acid* in the liver and to a lesser degree in the muscles and adipose (fat) tissue. Fatty acid manufactured in the liver will be transported via the blood stream and deposited in the adipose tissue and stored as *fat*. The more carbohydrates the patient eats, the more fat will be formed. The pre-adipocytes can continue to multiply to handle any extra amount of fatty acid produced. Now the patient's weight and waist circumference begins to increase. The patient starts as slightly overweight, and then slightly obese. The fasting blood glucose becomes slightly higher than normal, e.g. 6.5 mmol/L. This condition is called *impaired fasting glucose (IFG or pre-diabetic)*. The body is trying to maintain the blood glucose below the normal level of 5.6 mmol/L by increasing the secretion of insulin. This causes hyperinsulinemia, which may not be a good thing. Yes, the extra amount of insulin can lower the blood glucose level, but at the same time, it causes fat accumulation.

As the patient continues to overeat, even the extra insulin cannot handle the excessive amount of glucose in the blood (relative hypoinsulinemia). The fasting blood glucose level becomes higher than 7 mmol/L, and the patient is now labeled as diabetic. At this time, the Beta cells in the pancreas cannot produce enough insulin to meet the demand. This is called *Beta cell dysfunction*. It takes a few years for the obese non-diabetic patient to develop an impaired fasting glucose and glucose intolerance, and a few more years before the patient develops Type 2 diabetes. Once you become a diabetic, the Beta cell function will continue to deteriorate, even with medications. It is of vital importance to stop the conversion at the earliest stage so that the Beta cell function can be preserved. The only effective way to stop the conversion is to make an early diagnosis and to start aggressive lifestyle modification as soon as possible. There is evidence that with weight reduction, the Beta cell function improves in the pre-diabetic stage. *Prevention is much more effective than treatment.* The failure to diagnose impaired glucose tolerance is a missed opportunity to prevent the development of diabetes through lifestyle interventions. Hence, it was proposed that patients with a fasting blood glucose more than 5.6 mmol/L should be diagnosed as impaired fasting glucose, and should therefore be counseled and monitoring closely. At the time that this book was written, Canada used 6 mmol/L as the cut off point for the upper limit of normal blood glucose. You can stop 58% of patients with an impaired fasting glucose or impaired glucose tolerance from progressing to Type 2 diabetes with a 5% weight reduction[1-2]. The key is fat weight reduction. The question is how? Obese Type 2 diabetics have more difficulty in losing weight than obese individuals who do not have diabetes[3]. It does not make sense to treat the obese diabetic patient with medications like insulin and glyburide (Diabeta®), which promote weight gain.

Free fatty acids are elevated in most obese Type 2 diabetics, which suggest that free fatty acids themselves might induce hyperglycemia. Constant infusion of fatty acid in a test subject longer than 2 hours reduces insulin-mediated muscle glucose uptake and increases hepatic glucose output[4-5].

Table 3. Interpretation of the Screening Test Result for Diabetes (International Diabetic Federation).

Diagnosis	Fasting blood glucose	2-hour glucose tolerance test with 75 gram sugar load
Normal	<5.6 mmol/L	< 7.8 mmol/L
Impaired Fasting Glucose	5.7 - 6.9 mmol/L	< 7.8 mmol/L
Impaired Glucose Tolerance (Pre-diabetic)	5.7 - 6.9 mmol/L	7.8 - 11.0 mmol/L
Diabetes	> 7.0 mmol/L	> 11.0 mmol/L

In order to develop impaired fasting glucose (IFG), there has to be a decrease in the production of insulin in addition to insulin resistance. In impaired glucose tolerance (IGT), only peripheral insulin resistance is needed to produce abnormal results. IGT occurs before IFG. Hence, IGT is a better screening test than IFG. For patients with impaired fasting glucose or impaired glucose tolerance, lifestyle modification reduces the risk of dysglycemia and progression towards established diabetes mellitus[1].

The risk of developing coronary heart disease is doubled in patients with IGT when compared with normal patients. The risk became four fold if the patient has diabetes. Two thirds of patients with coronary heart disease have abnormal glucose metabolism[6].

The exact mechanism of how obesity causes diabetes is still unknown. The current thinking is that the development of Type 2 diabetes in the obese patient is due to the over production of circulating free fatty acid from the adipose tissue. The excessive amount of free fatty acid induces *insulin resistance*. For patients with insulin resistance, the muscle, liver, and adipose tissue do not respond to insulin as they usually do. Insulin resistance was originally defined as a state in which greater than normal amounts of insulin are required to elicit a quantitatively normal response. Later, it was proposed that insulin resistance existed when normal concentrations of insulin produced a less than normal biological response.

The Adiponectin level in the blood correlates well with insulin sensitivity. It inhibits platelet aggregation and functions as an anti-inflammatory agent. Its level is found to be low in the obese patients. In extremely obese women, gastric-bypass surgery induced weight loss increases adiponectin subcutaneous adipose tissue gene expression and plasma concentrations[7].

The major role of insulin is to promote the influx of glucose from the blood stream into the muscle cells. Glucose can be used up during routine daily activities or converted into glycogen for storage. For patients with insulin resistance, this transportation mechanism becomes weakened, and blood glucose has difficulty in moving into the muscle cells. The ability of insulin to promote glycogenesis (manufacture glycogen) in the muscle is also dampened. Hence, the blood glucose stays high in the blood and the glycogen storage in the muscle is low. The extra glucose is now available to form fat in muscle and adipocytes.

The same transportation mechanism fails in the liver, whereby glucose is not moving into the liver cells effectively. Instead, the free fatty acid that is found in abundance in the blood has a better chance to move into the liver cells instead. Insulin usually suppresses gluconeogenesis in the liver cells. With insulin resistance, liver manufactures glucose from glycerol and amino acids. This raises the blood glucose. When fatty acid gets stored as fat in the liver, it causes fatty liver.

Remember that one of the functions of insulin is to facilitate the movement of blood glucose into the cells, especially the liver, muscle, and fat cells. Consider the cell as a room with many doors. If all the doors are closed, glucose cannot enter inside the room. Insulin is like the key to these doors. It opens the doors and allows the glucose to go inside. The technical term for the doors is *insulin receptors*. Different types of cells contain different numbers of insulin receptors (doors) on the cell surface. It varies from less than 50 in the blood, brain or kidney cell to over 20,000 in the liver, muscle or fat cell. The more receptors there are on the cells, the bigger the influence of insulin. Since red blood, brain and kidney cells have only a small amount of insulin receptors, they do not rely on insulin for the transportation of glucose into the cells. This means that regardless of the amount of insulin present, glucose can still enter inside the blood, brain and kidney cells. In contrast, a normal amount of insulin must be present in order for glucose to enter the liver, muscle and fat cells.

Two major problems can occur with the receptors that prevent glucose from entering the cells.

1. The number of receptors on the cell surface can be reduced by the presence of an excessive amount of circulating insulin, as in hyperinsulinemia, secondary to obesity and/or glucose intolerance. Hence, there are fewer "doors" available for the glucose to enter the cells. This defect is reversible when hyperinsulinemia is corrected. An inherited problem with the receptor site is rare.

2. Even when insulin is able to bind to the receptor site, the glucose may still have problems entering the cell, as in the case of the Type 2 diabetic. Once this problem sets in, it cannot be corrected even with medications. The exact mechanism is not been fully understood yet. It was proposed that the free fatty acid is competing with the glucose at the same receptor site and so blocks the glucose molecule from getting into the cell.

In clinical practice, it is very difficult for the doctor to screen for insulin resistance. However, if the doctor can identify a patient suffering from insulin resistance before the patient becomes glucose intolerant or diabetic, the doctor can start treatment and avoid future complications. An indirect method to detecting insulin resistance consists of measuring the patient's fasting glucose and fasting insulin level. The following result may occur (providing the patient is not on any anti-diabetic medication).

Table 4. Interpretation of Fasting Glucose and Insulin Values.		
Fasting Glucose	Fasting Insulin	Interpretation
Low	Low	Non-diabetic Non-insulin resistance
Normal	Low	Non-diabetic Non-insulin resistance
High	Low	Diabetic, Beta cell dysfunction
Low	High	Non-diabetic Insulin secreting tumor
Normal	High	Pre-diabetic Insulin resistance
High	High	Diabetic, Insulin resistance, Beta cell dysfunction

An elevated fasting insulin to glucose ratio signifies insulin resistance. Insulin resistance is a pre-requisite to Type 2 diabetes. Dr. Gerald Schulman, professor on internal medicine and cellular and molecular physiology at the Yale University School of Medicine stated that insulin resistance is the best predictor of whether someone will eventually develop Type 2 diabetes. It is this pre-diabetic group who has a normal fasting glucose level but has a high insulin level that the doctor would like to identify. With appropriate treatment of this group of patients can revert back to normal glucose tolerance and avoid deterioration of the Beta cells. The drawback of this method is the inability to measure insulin levels accurately. There is no standardized testing method to measure insulin, and many laboratories have different "normal ranges". This makes it difficult to interpret the results. Most methods measure not only the insulin level but also the proinsulin level (lack of specificity). However, if the fasting insulin level is grossly elevated, then it is likely outside of the normal range. The following is a mathematic model used to assess insulin resistance. Homeostatic Model Assessment of Insulin Resistance index (HOMA-RI) is calculated by multiplying fasting insulin by fasting glucose and dividing by 22.5. The higher is the index, the higher is the insulin resistance.

Homeostatic Model Assessment of Insulin Resistance index (HOMA-RI)	
Percentile	HOMA-RI
10	1.1
25	1.4
50	2.3
75	2.6
90	4.1

Insulin is produced by the Beta cells situated in the pancreatic islets. It starts as a pro-insulin molecule inside the Beta cells and separates into insulin and C-peptide molecules in a 1:1 ratio before entering the blood stream. The liver will pick up about 40% of the released insulin. However, the liver will not remove any C-peptide molecules. Hence, measuring the C-peptide level in the blood is a more sensitive index than measuring the serum insulin level when assessing the Beta cell function (figure 3).

Figure 3. Production of Insulin in the Beta Cell.

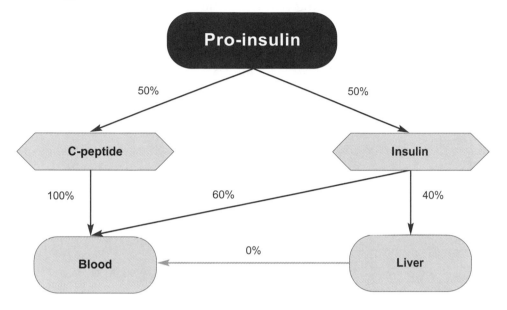

A spike of insulin is released into the portal circulation within 10 minutes of food intake; this is followed by a slower and more prolonged phase of insulin release that lasts up to 2 hours. The first phase of insulin secretion inhibits hepatic glucose production, while the second phase promotes glucose uptake by the peripheral tissues. For the obese Type 2 diabetic patient suffering from insulin resistance, the first phase of insulin release is lost and the second phase is impaired.

Before starting an obese Type 2 diabetic patient on insulin, the doctor can measure the patient's insulin level to see if indeed they require extra insulin. One critic noted that there is no accurate reference method in measuring insulin and different laboratory employs different methodologies. However, we feel that the absolute value is not of concern. As long as the patient is producing some insulin, the patient should be able to achieve glycemic control by losing weight with the appropriate diet. If the patient is taking insulin already, the doctor can measure C-peptide levels. Measuring the insulin level when the patient is already taking insulin will yield a result that is difficult to interpret because you cannot distinguish whether the insulin measured is coming from the pancreas or coming from the injections.

Insulin usually promotes the formation of triglycerides (fat) in adipose tissue. With insulin resistance, the adipose tissue oxidizes triglycerides, which is composed of one glycerol molecule and three fatty acid molecules, and liberates the fatty acid into the blood stream causing an elevated amount of free fatty acid in the blood. Indeed, most of the obese Type 2 diabetic patients do have a high level of free fatty acid in their blood. One theory about the cause of obesity induced insulin resistance is that the overproduction of free fatty acid competes with glucose as the preferred fuel of choice, causing an increase in the blood glucose level. Research found that when the circulating free fatty acid decreases, insulin sensitivity improves. This is why a Type 2 diabetic should decrease the consumption of fat. However, we did not say "no" fat at all. A certain amount of *essential fatty acid* intake is needed daily for health maintenance. Indeed, it was found that insulin sensitivity could be influenced by your diet. A diet that is high in saturated fat decreases insulin sensitivity, whereas a diet rich in monounsaturated fat promotes insulin sensitivity.

It has been known for a long time that fat accumulation in the abdomen called *central obesity* (or *visceral*, *truncal*, or *android obesity*), is closely associated with Type 2 diabetes, coronary heart disease and hyperuricemia. This type of fat only corresponds with 10 to 15% of total body fat. However, when you lose weight, 30% of the fat loss will be coming from the abdominal area. This is a good thing since this type of fat is pathological. Adiponectin is a hormone produced by the adipose cell. In normal weight and non-diabetic patients, adiponectin improves glucose uptake by the skeletal muscle cells and reduces gluconeogenesis (production of glucose by muscle and fat cells) in the liver cells. Hence, it increases insulin sensitivity and has a protective effect against diabetes. However, for some reason, the production of adiponectin by the adipose cell is blunted in the obese and Type 2 diabetic individuals[8-9]. The level of adiponectin can be increased with the use of thiazolidinediones (e.g. Actose® and Avandia®)[10], which enhance this class of drug can enhance insulin sensitivity and inhibit gluconeogenesis.

Another important risk factor that cannot be ignored is family history. If you have a first-degree relative (father, mother, brother, sister, child) with Type 2 diabetes and obesity, your chance of developing the same disease is increased, especially if you are gaining fat weight.

Dawn Phenomenon

In Type 2 diabetics, basal glucagon secretion is increased, which contributes to fasting hyperglycemia by increasing fasting hepatic glucose output. Glucagon suppression is blunted by hyperglycemia, especially when insulin levels are low. Insulin treatment does not reduce glucagon levels, however, and it is possible that the alpha cells in people with Type 2 diabetes may also contribute to insulin resistance. One of the normal functions of insulin is to prevent the breakdown of fat storage. During the insulin resistant state, fat cells in the abdominal area are particularly more resistant than the fat cells in the rest of the body. Hence, more fat is metabolized (lipolysis) in this area, and the fatty acid molecules released from the fat cells will go to the liver via a special blood circulation pathway (portal circulation). The liver cells are also prone to insulin resistance, which increases the rate of gluconeogenesis, and transforms part of the triglycerides molecule generated from fat cell breakdown into glucose. This is why the blood glucose level is elevated during the insulin resistant state, the glucose intolerant state or the diabetic state. In a non-diabetic healthy person who has no insulin resistance, the fasting blood sugar level is usually the lowest reading when compared to the blood glucose levels for the rest of the day.

The production of glucose by the liver occurs 24 hours a day in patients suffering from Type 2 diabetes with insulin resistance. Sometimes, blood glucose levels can even increase during sleep. This is called the

Dawn Phenomenon. During the daytime, you can burn off the extra glucose produced by the liver with activities (e.g. housework). However, your activities during sleep are at a minimum and therefore the extra glucose produced will not be utilized. As long as the fasting blood glucose is not excessively high, the Dawn Phenomenon may not be a bad thing.

One hypothesis behind the Dawn Phenomenon is that it is a biochemical adaptation that the human body has evolved which has allowed the human race to survive all these years. When the body senses that you have too much fat, especially in the abdominal area, it induces insulin resistance and stops the formation of more fat (lipogenesis). Through lipolysis of the fat cell and gluconeogenesis in the liver (and a small amount in the kidney), the body can lose fat weight. If you do not consume extra calories or excess carbohydrates and/or fat, your body should be able to continue to burn fat until you are no longer obese. Insulin resistance will disappear once you return to a healthy weight. We found that with the Dawn Phenomenon, the fasting blood glucose is only about 1 to 2 mmol/L higher than prior to sleep. If you can keep your nighttime glucose on the low side, the fasting blood glucose should still be acceptable. Hence, we encourage our patients to do some walking or exercise after their dinner in order to lower their blood glucose before going to bed. During exercise, muscle cells deplete their glucose and glycogen stores and will "suck-in" more glucose from the blood, hence lowering the blood glucose level. This is one of the mechanisms to fight insulin resistance in the muscle. Do not worry that your blood glucose will decrease during sleep. The glucose that causes the rise in fasting blood sugar is produced in vivo (from within) rather than in vitro (from outside). Cortisol is a type of hormone that is produced by the adrenal cortex. It causes mobilization of carbohydrates and fat and leads to an increase in blood glucose. Since the cortisol level highest when we wake up in morning, the fasting glucose level may be higher at this time.

The goal of treatment when dealing with an obese Type 2 diabetic patient is to lose the fat weight. In a way, insulin resistance and Dawn Phenomenon have assisted the patient in achieving this goal. This is what we call "burn fat while you sleep". In our experience, this transient elevation of blood glucose will not affect the A1c, an average of blood glucose levels over a period of three months. Hence, it does not increase the risk of diabetic complications, as long as the blood glucose is under control for the rest of the day. The Dawn Phenomenon may be used as indirect evidence of the presence of insulin resistance.

If a patient is given higher carbohydrate meals throughout the day, blood glucose and fasting blood glucose increase. If the doctor give this patient some medication such as glyburide, Diamicron®, Starlix®, Amaryl®, or GlucoNorm® (which indirectly promote the secretion of more insulin), or insulin injections, this extra insulin will bring down the blood glucose. However, the extra insulin also stops the fat burning by inhibiting gluconeogenesis and actually promotes lipogenesis! This is why it is of utmost importance that obese patients with insulin resistance to limit carbohydrate intake, and to let the body burn off fat naturally. Some experts say that you need to consume carbohydrate everyday because your body needs glucose to function. We agree. However, if you have so much glucose stored in abdominal fat and you can produce glucose and energy from burning that adipose tissue, why bother eating extra sugar. Are you saving that fat for future use, such as famine?

Patients with Type 2 diabetes but are on insulin injections find it very difficult to lose weight. Hence, in order to help these patients to lose weight, one should try to wean the patient off insulin as soon as possible (without sacrificing the glycemic control). Ensure that the patient produces enough insulin by doing a C-peptide test. This diet has the ability to lower the blood glucose level and therefore allows the patient to decrease gradually the insulin dose as the blood glucose level decreased. This drop in blood glucose value can occurs within a few days after started on the diet. Patients should be warned ahead of time to watch out for hypoglycemia (low blood sugar). Do glucometer readings before giving insulin injections. A sliding scale should be given to the patient. If the value is below 7 mmol/L, the dose of insulin should be decreased by 30-50%. If the value is below 6 mmol/L, the dose should be decreased by 50-70%. If the value is below 5 mmol/L, no insulin should be given. Once the insulin dose is decreased, you do not have to increase the insulin dose even if the blood glucose is slightly higher the next day. Just stick to the diet, the blood glucose will come down again once you lose more weight. Continue to lower the insulin requirement as the blood glucose level decreases until the patient is off insulin completely. Adjust the oral anti-diabetic medications as needed. If you are a patient, *do not adjust the insulin dose yourself.* Ask the medical professional to do it for you. Your family doctor needs to monitor you very closely to make sure that you are doing it correctly and safely.

Another common "complication" that patients experience is blurry vision, which occurs when the blood glucose returns to near normal from poorly controlled diabetes. Do not be alarmed, as it might be a good complication. When the blood glucose is constantly elevated in a poorly controlled diabetic, glucose enters the lens of the eyes, drawing in water at the same time. This leads to swelling of the lens. The brain has the ability to adapt to this spherical lens curvature and you can see things relatively clearly, although this lens shape can increase the risk of glaucoma. As your blood glucose returns to normal, glucose will leave the lens and return to the blood stream. Water will also move out of the lens and therefore restores the normal lens curvature. It will take a few days for your brain to re-adjust to the normal shaped lens. If you have experience blurry vision as your blood glucose improves, do not panic. Usually only the near vision is affected, and therefore your driving should not be impaired. Your vision will return to normal after a few days to a week of adjustment.

Patients who are dependant on insulin, even if they are Type 2 diabetic to begin with, will not be able to wean off insulin completely. However, they can still benefit from this diet by being able to lower the insulin requirement and achieve better glycemic control. Again, do not adjust the insulin dose yourself without the approval of your medical supervisor.

The abnormally high level of blood glucose in the Type 2 diabetic patient can result from:

1. Overconsumption of carbohydrates, and/or

2. The inability of insulin to move glucose from the blood (insulin resistance) to the target organs (liver, muscle, and adipose tissue) and/or

3. The over production of glucose from glycerol or amino acids by the liver (gluconeogenesis), and/or

4. Pancreatic burn out (Beta cell dysfunction) in which the pancreas can no longer catch up with the demand for more insulin production and/or

5. Taking medications that promote hyperglycemia (Table 5)

In order to normalize the blood glucose level of these patients, one needs to tackle all the five points listed above at the same time. This diet plan is low in carbohydrates, fulfilling the requirement of item number 1. Taking anti-diabetic medications can only solve half of the problems listed in items number 2 and 3. Regular exercise can help with the other half. Exercise can improve insulin sensitivity and drives the blood glucose into the cells. The Da Qing study in China demonstrated that with exercise and diet, one could reduce the risk of converting impaired glucose tolerance to diabetes by 31 to 58%. Once the pancreas is burned out, you have no choice but to take insulin by injection. A Type 2 diabetic should avoid taking thiazide diuretics, non-selective beta-blockers, prednisone, antipsychotic or high-dose contraceptives if the blood glucose is not well-controlled. However, if you have to take these types of medication due to other medical reasons, by all means, go ahead. You can still lose weight by working harder on other parts of the diet plan.

Diabetic medications should be used to control the blood glucose levels until the diet and exercise starts to take effect. Do not stop your medications without the physician's knowledge. It was suggested that if the A1c (a blood test that shows your blood glucose over the past three months) is over 9%, one should start taking two anti-diabetic medications immediately.

A few words of caution about the A1c blood test. It is *not* a screening test for diabetes. As stated above, it is the average of your blood glucose over two to three months. If your blood glucose is under control most of the time and only occasionally high because of partying your A1c will be normal. This A1c test has one major limitation. Its result is invalid if you have abnormal hemoglobin, like hemoglobin S (sickle cell), hemoglobin C, thalassemia, etc. Especially if there is a family history of unexplainable anemia, there is a possibility of abnormal hemoglobin, even if it is not detectable with hemoglobin electrophoresis. A1c should be used to follow the patient's progress instead of as a diagnostic tool. Patients that are suffering from iron, vitamin B12, folate deficiency, anemia, or end stage renal disease may also have an elevated A1c even if the blood glucose is under good control.

Table 5. Drugs that can Potentially Worsen Blood Glucose Control.

Drugs	Possible Mechanisms
Propranolol (Inderal LA®)	Inhibit insulin secretion Increase insulin resistance Alter lipid metabolism
Thiazide diuretics (less common for Lasix® or Lozide®)	Decrease insulin secretion Increase insulin resistance
Salbutamol (Ventolin®) Terbutaline (Bricanyl®)	Increase glycolysis (utilization of glucose) Increase glycogenolysis Increase insulin resistance
Niacin (lipid-lowering agent)	Increase free fatty acid
Clozapine (Clozaril®) Risperidone (Risperdal®) Olanzapine (Zyprexa®)	Weight gain Lipid abnormalities
Prednisone (Corticosteroids)	Decrease insulin sensitivity Increase gluconeogenesis Increase lipolysis Enhance glucagon secretion

Management of Type 2 diabetes may require a combination of lifestyle modification and medications. Table 6 illustrates the different methods in treatment of patients with Type 2 diabetes. For example, one of the goals is to decrease glucose intake in order to achieve glycolysis, lipolysis and gluconeogenesis. The method used to achieve this goal is to eat a low-carbohydrate diet. Another treatment goal is to decrease circulating free fatty acids in order to reduce insulin resistance through eating a low-carbohydrate-low-fat diet and/or taking Xenical®.

Table 6. Treatment Options for Type 2 Diabetes.

Goals	To Achieve	Methods
Decrease glucose intake	Lipolysis	Low-carb diet
Decrease free fatty acid in blood	Reduction of insulin resistance	Low-carb-low-fat diet, Xenical®
Increase insulin sensitivity	Reduction of hyperinsulinemia	Exercise, Low-carb-low-fat diet, Metformin
Increase lipolysis	Reduction of total body-fat	Low-carb-low-fat diet, Magnesium supplement
Increase glucose utilization	Better glycemic (blood sugar) control	Exercise, Build up muscle mass
Preserve Beta cell function	Preservation of insulin production	Actose®, Avandia® Low-carb-low-fat diet
Prevent co-mobidities	Blood pressure control, Maintenance of normal renal function, Normal lipid profile, Cardioprotection, Normal coagulation profile	Exercise, Low-sodium diet, ACEs, e.g. Altace® ARBs, e.g. Avapro®, Statins, e.g. Lipitor®, Aspirin
Increase insulin level in blood	Better glycemic control	Diabeta®, Diamicron®, GlucoNorm®, Amaryl®, Starlix®
Slow down glucose absorption in gut	Lower postprandial (after meal) blood glucose elevation	Prandase®

Table 7 lists the most commonly used anti-diabetic medications. There are pros and cons associated with each group of medications. The choice of medication should be made according to the patient type.

Table 7. Pharmacological Agents used in the Treatment of Type 2 Diabetic.

Medication	Action	Side Effects	Usage
Insulin (Humulin®)	Promote the transfer of glucose into cells, increase glycogen and fat synthesis	Hypoglycemia (low blood sugar), low serum potassium, weight gain	Type 1 diabetic, Poorly controlled type 2 diabetic, pregnancy
Sulfonylurea (Diabeta®, Diamicron®), Repaglinide (GlucoNorm®), Nateglinide (Starlix®), Glimepiride (Amaryl®)	Increase insulin secretion	Hypoglycemia, intolerance to alcohol, weight gain, ineffective with pancreatic burn out	Good to use on type 2 diabetic who are thin and has low serum insulin or C-peptide level
Alpha-glucosidase inhibitor (Prandase®)	Delays digestion of carbohydrate, inhibits alpha-glucosidase	Bloating, diarrhea, need to monitor liver function	Decrease postprandial (after meal) hyperglycemia (high sugar)
Metformin (Glucophage®)	Decrease liver gluconeogenesis, decrease insulin resistance	Acidosis in patient with renal failure, diarrhea, need to monitor renal function	Decrease fasting glucose, weight loss, reduce circulating insulin, decrease insulin resistance
Piglitazone HCL (Actos®), Resiglitazone Maleate (Avandia®)	Decrease muscle and fat cell gluconeogenesis, decrease insulin resistance	Weight gain, peripheral edema, increase subcutaneous fat , heart failure, increase LDL and triglycerides, need to monitor liver function	Synergetic effect with metformin, reduce circulating insulin, preserve Beta cell function
Orlistat (Xenical®)	Inhibit Lipase, decrease free fatty acid	Oily spotting, diarrhea	Weight loss, improves glycemic control and lipid profile
Sibutramine (Meridia®)	Promote satiety, thermogenesis	Dry mouth, insomnia, increase heart rate and blood pressure, takes a long time to work	Suppress appetite, weight loss

The following passage was copied from the product information of Glimepiride (Amaryl®).

"Warning: use of Glimepiride must be considered as treatment in addition to a proper dietary regimen and not as a substitute for diet.... Over a period of time, patients may become progressively less responsive to therapy with oral hypoglycemic agents because of deterioration of their diabetic state."

All oral anti-diabetic medications are contraindicated during pregnancy. Insulin is the only one that has been proven safe to use. Some expects are now prescribing metformin during pregnancy and no adverse drug reactions have been reported yet. For the high-risk female who wishes to avoid gestational diabetes, she should try to maintain a healthy weight prior to conception. She must not gain more than 30 pounds during her pregnancy. Although there is no data to indicate that a mild maternal ketosis is harmful to the fetus, I would not advice expecting mothers to start this diet from Phase 1. She can follow the principle of the Phase 2 diet to control her weight gain during pregnancy.

If the patient is a Type 2 diabetic who is of slim built and has low serum insulin, sulfonylurea type medication is the drug of choice. Conversely, if the patient is obese and has hyperinsulinemia, sulfonylurea will be a bad choice. Biguanide (metformin) will be the drug of choice. There is a dose related adverse side effect of glyburide (Diabeta®) related to cardiovascular events. That is to say that when a patient with heart disease is started on glyburide, the chance of a heart attack is increased. The same relationship is not observed with metformin[11]. This implies that the manner in which blood glucose level is lowered may be as important as achieving recommended glucose targets.

If the blood glucose cannot be controlled with metformin alone, an insulin sensitizer like pioglitazone or rosiglitazone should be added. One word of caution for using this class of drug is that it can cause peripheral edema, weight gain, subcutaneous fat gain, and congestive heart failure. Hence both the American Diabetic Association and the

American Heart Association suggested that patients who are elderly (over 70 years old), with a history of congestive heart failure, hypertension, coronary heart disease, significant renal disease (creatinine more than 187 mol/L) or taking insulin, should avoid using this class of medication. The risk of developing lactate acidosis is elevated in this population. However, a review article written by McCormack et al concluded that the benefit outweigh the risk even in the high-risk group[12].

We have seen many instances when obese patients with Type 2 diabetes are prescribed with insulin because their blood sugar cannot be controlled with the usual oral medications. There are a few drawbacks with this type of treatment.

Firstly, these patients are already likely have hyperinsulinemia. This means that they are producing a lot of insulin, but because of insulin resistance and poor eating habits, they require more insulin to counteract the insulin resistance. By giving them more insulin, you are worsening their hyperinsulinemia. The hyperinsulinemia is causing complications with their obesity in the first place. However, the specialists did not believe in testing for fasting insulin or C-peptide levels to assess if the patients were producing normal amounts of insulin! If the patient can still produce some insulin on their own, one can treat the patient by lowering their insulin requirement (e.g. decrease fat weight, eat less sugar and carbohydrate, and do more exercise). Our research had found that 87% of our obese Type 2 diabetic patients who are taking insulin produce normal or extra amount of endogenous insulin[13.] Energy should be channeled to deal with the insulin resistance by a vigorous weight reduction through diet manipulation, an exercise program and oral insulin sensitizing medications. Giving extra in*sulin does not treat the insulin resistance.* On the other hand, if the patient has a very low insulin production, as shown by blood test, they have no choice but to start insulin injections. In this case, the insulin that is given will not produce hyperinsulinemia. It is simply a replacement of what the patient does not have. This type of patient is usually thin and/or normal weight and/or elderly, but not obese.

Secondly, dieticians at a diabetic clinic will give patients a set of instructions when they attend an insulin injection teaching class. Insulin injections may cause hypoglycemia (low blood sugar), which is a potentially life threatening reaction, and can be a very frightening experience. Therefore, patients are told to eat some carbohydrates before every injection. Some are told to eat half of a sandwich, a fruit or a few cookies before they go to bed to avoid hypoglycemia during sleep. What happens then is that the blood glucose increases after the ingestion of the carbohydrate-rich snack. Where does the blood glucose end up going? With the help of the insulin injection, the blood glucose gets transformed into fat and stored in the belly (gaining inches while you sleep)! This is why most patients gain weight after they are started on insulin. Imagine that some patients use four doses of insulin per day. This patient has to load up on carbohydrates at least four times a day with the insulin injections, on top of the carbohydrates from the regular meals.

Thirdly, insulin enhances a patient's appetite. They feel hungry all the time, which leads to overeating.

A common technique used by the diabetic clinic is called *carb counting*. In order to provide a tighter control of patient's blood sugar, the patients are told to give themselves a dose of rapidly acting insulin (e.g. Novolin Rapid®) just before their meals. The amount of insulin used depends on the amount of carbohydrates they are about to consume. The patients are taught to calculate the amount of carbohydrates in the meal and give themselves 1 unit of rapidly acting insulin per 10 to 12 grams of carbohydrates consumed. For example, John is about to eat a bowl of cereal with a glass of milk. He figures out that there is a total of 42 grams of carbohydrate in this meal, using the information printed on the boxes. He gives himself 4 units of insulin before he eats. The idea is that the blood glucose will not go up much because the insulin given should cover the ingested carbohydrates. However, if John happens to be obese and his glycogen storage spaces are full, the insulin is going to drive the carbohydrates into the fat cells, where they will be stored as fat! If John's meal contains very little to no carbohydrates, then there is no need to give himself any insulin before his meal to cover any potential post-meal blood glucose elevation and he will not gain fat weight. Remember, *insulin plus carbohydrates equal fat gain*. There is no such thing as protein counting because John's blood sugar will not go up even after he consumes a big egg white omelet. Eating protein does not lead to hyperglycemia[14-15]. Hence John does not have to give himself any insulin prior to eating the egg white omelet. As long as he does not eat sugar or starch, his own insulin production will be enough to maintain a normal blood glucose level.

Due to the fear of hypoglycemia, Type 2 diabetics who were prescribed with insulin had worse glycemic control. Patients intentionally kept their blood glucose high to prevent hypoglycemia[16]. The risk of severe hypoglycemia over a 6-year period was 2.4% with metformin, 3.3% with sulfonylurea and 11.2% with insulin[17].

With careful monitoring and counseling, we were able to wean patients off insulin and keep their blood glucose under excellent control. These patients are then able to lose weight faster in the absence of exogenous insulin.

According to the United Kingdom Prospective Diabetes Study (UKPDS)[17], most Type 2 diabetics end up requiring insulin 14 years after diagnosis. However, that study is dated. Newer studies, like the ACCORD, ADVANCE and VADT studies all demonstrated that the A1c can be controlled with aggressive treatment. Improvement of glycemic control leads to increased beta cell survival. The reverse is also true. Consistently high blood glucose increases the rate of beta cell apoptosis, a condition called *glucose toxicity*.

Experts suggested that patient start insulin early to prevent complications. Ninety percent of newly diagnosed Type 2 diabetics are obese and obesity is one of the hallmarks of insulin resistance. Most obese patients gain weight when started on insulin, which increases insulin resistance. Complications of Type 2 diabetes are known to have resulted from hyperinsulinemia. If the patient has a high endogenous insulin production, giving extra insulin can worsen the condition. We reviewed the charts of one hundred and thirty one obese Type 2 diabetic patients using insulin. The average age was 57, 44% were male, the average BMI was 38.6, and the average A1C was 8.4%[13]. The average number of years being diabetic was 15 and average number of years on insulin was 5.8. Serum C-peptide levels were measured on all 131 patients on their first visit. The normal range is 350 to 1650. Only 4 out of 131 patients (3%) produced almost no C-peptide. Thirteen patients (10%) had sub-optimal levels from 160 to 350. Ninety-four patients (71%) produced normal amounts of C-peptide, and twenty patients (16%) produced higher than normal levels of C-peptide (hyperinsulinemia). The majority of the obese Type 2 diabetics (87%) produced normal amounts of insulin, just not enough to counteract the insulin resistance caused by extra adipose tissue, or that their diet is too high in carbohydrate. Only 25% of patients achieved an A1c of 7% or less (4% achieved A1c of 6% or less), despite using insulin. Effort should be channelled into teaching lifestyle changes in order to fight insulin resistance, instead of starting the patient on insulin.

There are some newer types of oral anti-hyperglycemic medications (GlucoNorm®, Amaryl® and Starlix®) designed to help with controlling the postprandial rise in blood sugar. They have a fast onset of action. They induce insulin secretion from the pancreatic beta cells to cover the rise in blood glucose after a meal. Hence, to avoid postprandial hyperglycemia, the patient has to take the pill immediately before each meal. This type of medication has little use in this diet because this diet is very low in carbohydrates and does not require coverage to prevent hyperglycemia. If the patient takes GlucoNorm®, Amaryl® or Starlix®

before a low carbohydrate meal, the medications can actual induce hypoglycemia.

Acarbose (Glucobay®) is a new type of anti-diabetic agent known as an alpha-glucosidase inhibitor. This drug delays the digestion of ingested carbohydrates, thereby resulting in a smoothing and lowering of blood glucose concentration following meals. Consequently, acarbose lowers the patient's A1c. This acts like a "carb blocker". However, acarbose only "blocks" the absorption of starch and sucrose (fruits), but allows the absorption of maltose (beer) or lactose (milk) or monosaccharide such as fructose (e.g., fructose sweetened drinks). In addition, a liver function test is needed in the first 6 months to make sure that the drug did not affect the liver. Presented at the 18th International Diabetes Federation Congress in Paris, France, August 2003, postprandial blood glucose is more important than the fasting blood glucose in predicting complications. The two-hour postprandial blood glucose is an independent risk factor for cardiovascular disease regardless of fasting plasma glucose levels. Instead of worrying about this, why not decrease the amount of carbohydrates in the first place. The postprandial blood glucose will not go up if you are not eating carbohydrates if you have a high A1c of less than 8.5%, the postprandial glucose level is likely responsible for the increased A1c.

Postprandial hyperglycemia appears to be the rate-limiting factor for achieving optimal glycemic control in many patients with type 2 diabetes[18]. The objective of medical treatment is to keep the fasting glucose below 5.6 mmol/L, the two-hour post-prandial glucose below 8 mmol/L, and an A1c less than 6% (Table 8). Do not settle with just acceptable control. Always strive to achieve the optimal control to prevent complications. Co-morbid conditions such as hypertension and dyslipidemia also need to be treated.

The drug of choice for obese Type 2 diabetics is metformin. It helps patients to lose weight, increase insulin sensitivity, and suppress gluconeogenesis and elevated blood glucose levels. The risk of hypoglycemia is low. There are contraindications for using metformin in certain patient populations. According to the Compendium of Pharmaceuticals and Specialties, patients with renal impairment (serum creatinine over 136 mmol/L for men and 124 mmol/L for women), congestive heart failure and over the age of 80 should not be put on metformin. The risk of developing lactic acidosis is elevated in this population. However, a review article written by McCormack concluded that the benefit outweighed the risk even in the high-risk group[12].

It was found that the rate of development of diabetic complications (such as microvascular diseases of the eye, kidney and nerves) corresponds to the A1c level. Hence, it is very important to keep a tight control on blood glucose level. Even better is to prevent the development of diabetes in the first place. High-risk individuals (family history, obesity, gestational diabetes, and impaired glucose tolerance) should be identified early and counseled on the importance of lifestyle changes. Lifestyle changes, such as weight loss, diet, and physical activities have been shown to prevent the development of diabetes in these individuals. As the population ages, the total number of obese Type 2 diabetics is on the rise.

Most of the obese Type 2 diabetics develop high blood pressure years before developing diabetes. The choice of antihypertensive medication can make a difference in these patients. According to the Anglo-Scandinavian Cardiac Outcome Trial (ASCOT), patients using calcium channel blockers (CCB) and angiotensin converting enzyme (ACE) inhibitors have a less chance of developing Type 2 diabetes than with beta-blockers and diuretics[19]. They propose that there are four mechanisms for the diabetogenic effect of beta-blockers and diuretics.

1. Increase in insulin resistance in the liver and increase in gluconeogenesis.

2. Increase in peripheral vascular constriction and decrease in peripheral tissue profusion.

3. Impaired insulin secretion due to pancreatic beta-receptor blockage.

4. Effect on the actual receptor and post-receptor. Thiazide diuretics may produce a hypokelemic state, a decrease in insulin secretion and reduced insulin-receptor sensitivity.

It is also suggested that both beta-blockers and thiazide diuretics cause a slow down in a patient's metabolism through slowing the conversion of T4 to T3. Hence, patients become obese and develop further insulin resistance.

Case #1. When Mrs. FW joined our program, she was 48 years old. Her weight was 234 pounds, body mass index of 41, and 46 percent body fat (108 pounds of fat). She had been a Type 2 diabetic for many years. She had to take Starlix® 120 mg three times per day and metformin 1000 mg twice a day. At that time, her fasting blood sugar was 9.6 mmol/L and A1c was at 0.067 (6.7%), which indicated that she needed stricter diabetic control. Just 4 weeks into this diet program, without changing her medications, her fasting blood sugar lowered to 6.1 mmol/L. Her Starlix® was then lowered by one pill and she only had to take it twice a day. Her fasting urine consistently showed no urine sugar and was positive for ketones. This meant that she was in ketosis due to fat burning, and *not ketoacidosis* (see Chapter 8). As her weight came down and with better blood glucose control, her Starlix® was decreased to once a day. Then, after 2 months on this diet, it was discontinued. After 11 weeks on the diet, another set of blood work was completed. This time the A1c lowered to 0.055 (5.5%) indicating excellent sugar control. Her weight at this time was 193 pounds, a drop of 41 pounds. Her body mass index was 34.2, and her percent body fat was 43%. This equals to a drop of 25 pounds of fat. Hence, out of the 41 pounds of weight that she lost, 25 pounds were due to fat loss. This translates to 61% efficiency in burning fat. Patients who do more exercise and weight training will have an even better fat burning efficiency. Mrs. FW does not exercise at all. She continues to take metformin to control her diabetes. Her husband, Mr. JW was 301 pounds when he started on the same diet at the same time. He was taking Diovan® 80 mg daily for hypertension. After two months on the diet, he lost 33 pounds and his blood pressure dropped to 105/72. Diovan® was discontinued. After another two months and another 21 pounds of weight loss (247 pounds), his blood pressure was maintained at 108/78 without medications.

Case #2. People should know that once you are diabetic, you will be diabetic for life, as there is no cure for this disease. The best one can do is to get the blood glucose under control without medications. If the diabetes has been long standing and the pancreas fails to produce enough insulin, the likelihood to stopping insulin or oral medications will be very minimal. However, for the obese patient who has just started to become diabetic, a simply lifestyle change can be enough to control the disease. Using Mrs. MC as an example, her diabetes is in excellent control because she does not have to take medications and her blood glucose is normal. She used to take Diabeta® twice a day. If she continues with the low-carbohydrate-low-fat-low-sodium diet for life, and does not regain her weight, her diabetes will not return.

Table 8. Target Values for Patient with Diabetes.

Recommended Targets for Sugar Control			
	A1c	**Fasting Sugar**	**2-Hour After Eating**
Target	< 0.070	4.0 - 7.0	5.0 - 10.0
Optimal	< 0.060	4.0 - 5.6	5.0 - 8.0
Recommended Targets for Lipids			
	LDL	**HDL**	**TC/HDL Ratio**	**Triglycerides**
Target	<3.5	>1.0	<5.0	<1.5
Optimal	<2.5	>1.0	<4.0	<1.0
Recommended Targets for Blood Pressure		
Target	130/80
Optimal	120/80

Case #3. Mrs. ES's diabetic condition posed a challenge. She is 52 years old and a Type 2 diabetic on insulin because her diabetes could not be controlled with the usual oral anti-diabetic medications. She was using 25 units of Humalog® mix and two grams of metformin per day. Her fasting glucose was 8 mmol/L. Since insulin could cause her to gain fat weight and defeat the purpose of this diet, my first objective was to get her sugar under better control. Then we lowered the dosage of her insulin aggressively. I started her on my diet and I warned her that she had to monitor her blood glucose very closely because her blood glucose came down very quickly. Within one week, her glucometer readings came down to an average of 7 mmol/L. She experienced a few episodes of hypoglycemia (low blood sugar) where she had to take some sugar tablets. Taking sugar tablets (carbohydrate) frequently for hypoglycemia will defeat the purpose of this diet. Hence, her insulin dosage was lowered immediately. We would rather see a slightly higher blood sugar value than one that is too low. Her urine was negative for both sugar and ketone bodies. We did not expect a lot of ketosis because one of the functions of insulin is to prevent fat burning (liposis). Therefore, it was important to eliminate her insulin injections entirely and as soon as possible. She stayed in Phase 1 (see Chapter 15) of the diet most of the time. After 12 weeks, she lost 22 pounds (from 225 pounds to 203 pounds) and she did not have to use insulin anymore. Her A1c came down to 0.060. She was maintained on two grams of metformin per day and even after 1 year, her A1c was still below 0.060.

It is very important that Type 2 diabetics on medications are under the strictest supervision of a physician before attempting this diet. Do not reduce your medications on your own. A patient with end stage Type 2 diabetes (low serum insulin, high urine sugar and ketones) will require the use of insulin and should not be on this diet. This type of patient can no longer produce enough insulin even while taking medications to boost insulin production.

According to the United Kingdom Prospective Diabetes Study (UKPDS)[20-22], a drawback in the treatment of Type 2 diabetes is that despite the availability of different oral anti-diabetic agents and insulin, the A1c level continues to get worse with time (Figure 4). This is to say that once you become diabetic, even if your A1c is under good control for the time being (by taking anti-diabetic medications), your A1c is going to get worse with time and you will require more medications to keep the A1c under control. It will come to a point that you will require insulin and eventually have to increase the insulin to get to the desirable result. Doctors seldom mention this to their diabetic patients. Medical doctors may not know how to counsel patients to prevent and/or slow down the deterioration of glycemic control. This book will show you later that the conclusion made by this study may not be correct.

Figure 4. Deterioration of A1c Even with Medications.

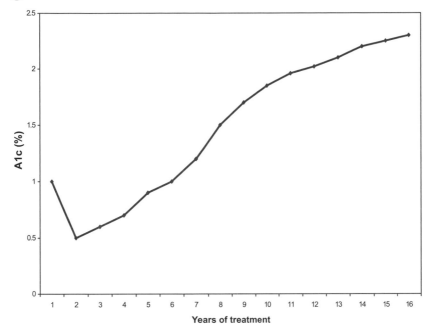

(Adopt from UKPDS Study)

Deterioration of glycemic control in Type 2 diabetics may be caused by:

1. Beta-cell burnout (Figure 5). There is about a 40% loss in the Beta-cell function once the patient is diagnosed with Type 2 diabetes. UKPDS shows that this deterioration continues even with aggressive medical therapy

2. Side effects of certain anti-diabetic medications, e.g. the insulin secretagogues (Diabeta®, Diamicron®, GlucoNorm®, Starlix®, Amaryl®)

3. Chronic hyperinsulinemia

4. Chronic hyperglycemia (Glucotoxicity)[23]

5. High circulating free fatty acids (Lipotoxicity)[23]

The exact mechanism is not known yet. It is likely caused by multiple factors. Progressive hyperglycemia will worsen Type 2 diabetes secondary to glucotoxicity. Short-term mild hyperglycemia enhances the insulin response to hyperglycemia[24]. Long-term mild hyperglycemia and short-term severe hyperglycemia dulls the insulin response[25]. Marked accumulation of lipids within islets impairs insulin secretion.

In insulin sensitive cells, such as liver, muscle and fat cells, the surface receptor is call Glucose Transporter 4 (GLUT4). GLUT4 requires insulin to function properly. Fatty acids compete with glucose to bind GLUT4, thereby producing insulin resistance. Other cells, like the brain cell, consist mainly GLUT 1, 2 and 3, and only a very little amount of GLUT4. Hence, these cells do not rely on insulin for glucose transport.

Fatty acids produce many Acetyl Co-A molecules through beta-oxidation, and overwhelmed the Kreb (Tricarboxylic Acid) Cycle. With the increase of ATP and citrate, phosphofructokinase, an enzyme for glycolysis, is inhibited. Thus, glycolysis is slowed down, inducing hyperglycemia. Fatty acids might decrease glucose conversion into glycogen for storage, thereby increasing the chance of hyperglycemia[26]. The opposite is also true. High levels of glucose produce a high level of Acetyl Co-A. Acetyl Co-A is then converted to malonyl Co-A, which is a potent inhibitor of carrier-mediated transport into mitochondria; it mediates glucose inhibition of fat oxidation. This means that fat burning is slowed down. Malonyl Co-A is the first step of fatty acid synthesis in the cytosol, which subsequently produces triglycerides. It is important to understand that the main cause of high serum triglycerides in the obese patient is not from overconsumption of fat but is rather due to the over intake of sugar and starch.

Sympathetic nervous system activation causes lipolysis, which increases in free fatty acids and increases in insulin resistance. Avoid stress, sleep deprivation and obesity, which activate the sympathetic nervous system. Weight reduction decreases the sympathetic tone.

All of the above points indicate that a diet high in sugar, starch and fat is bad for glucose metabolism. However, protein has never been implicated in diabetes. There is no such thing as protein toxicity. Protein actually improves glycemic control through the mechanism mentioned above. When the meal is of protein only, there is no change in the post-meal blood glucose level. In the fed state, the amino acids from the digested proteins that will go to the liver, which will convert the amino acids to proteins to repair our bodies and replace our daily obligatory protein loss. Any extra amino acids will be stored as glycogen and fat. When the blood glucose is low, as in the fasting state, amino acids and protein form the muscle can be mobilized to convert into glucose to provide energy for our bodily functions. This conversion is a very slow process. Remember, protein will only convert into glucose if the blood glucose is low. In the diabetic patient with either normal or high blood glucose levels, the conversion of protein into glucose will not take place and does not produce hyperglycemia postprandially. The ingested protein will be converted into muscle, glycogen or fat, in this specific order. It is a well-known fact that when patient who is taking insulin is suffering from low blood glucose, the patient is to drink juice so that the blood glucose can be raised quickly. We tell the patient not to try to raise the blood glucose by eating a piece of meat because we know that that piece of meat will not raise the blood glucose. This means that if you do not wish to raise your blood glucose after a meal, the best thing to eat is protein.

We do not believe that deterioration of the beta cell function is inevitable. In fact, studies using the newer type of oral anti-diabetic medications showed that they can prevent beta cell deterioration. The UKPDS study, which was done over 15 years ago, claims that glycemic control and beta cell function in a Type 2 diabetic will continue to deteriorate regardless of treatment type (e.g. Diabeta®, metformin, or night time insulin), the glycemic control and beta cell function will continue to deteriorate. It also found that the study subjects were not able to lose weight (using their dietary counseling). Did anyone ask why the patients were no able to lose weight? What kind of diet plan were they on? Is their blood glucose deterioration secondary to the fact that they are on the wrong diet? I have been to many diabetic conferences where the endocrinologists, diabetic educators and dietitians consistently quote this study and concluded that dietary treatment and oral medications will not work. Their suggestion is to prescribe the patient with multiple doses of insulin as soon as possible. They suggested that progressive deterioration is genetic, and that there is nothing the patient can do to alter the inevitable. We think that they are missing the boat. Result from our clinics have demonstrated that when patients follow this diet, not only will they lose weight, but the blood glucose will be better controlled, leading to a stable A1c level and prevents beta cell deterioration. Most of the time, medications will have to be adjusted downward to avoid hypoglycemia. If patient's beta cells are still functioning, the patient may even go off insulin and continue to have well-controlled blood glucose. The reason that the subjects in the UKPDS study did poorly with their glycemic control may not be due to failed medications, but rather a failed diet. Treatment of Type 2 diabetes is through weight reduction, diet and exercise, and not with medication. *Medication only treats the numbers; weight reduction treats the cause.* Studies using the newer type of oral anti-diabetic medications showed that they can prevent beta cell deterioration, contradicting the conclusion of the UKPDS study.

Figure 5. Deterioration of Beta Cell Function.

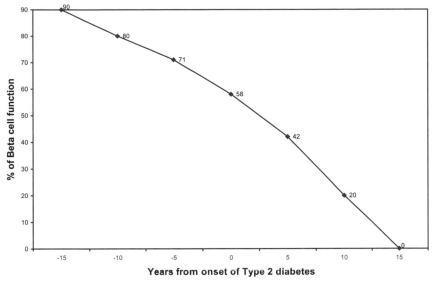

Years from onset of Type 2 diabetes

(According to the UKPDS Study)

Using a multi-faceted approach, we propose the following treatment strategies.

1. Decrease the requirement of insulin by decreasing the amount of carbohydrate intake and eat food with a low glycemic index (i.e. low glycemic load, see Chapter 11). If your body does not have to over work the beta cells, they may last longer. Moderate amounts of exercise increases the number of insulin receptors and makes the receptors more sensitive to insulin thus decreasing hyperinsulinemia. Free fatty acids will also decrease when the body fat percentage returns to normal with weight reduction. Weight loss therapy concomitantly improves beta cell function, lowers plasma glucagon concentrations, and improves insulin action in obese older adults[27].

2. Discontinue the use of insulin secretagogues (Diabeta®, Diamicron®, GlucoNorm®, Starlix®, Amaryl®) as soon as the glucose is under control. The use of insulin secretagogues is like

squeezing toothpaste out of the tube. There is a transient increase in the secretion of insulin, but eventually it becomes dry. When a patient has poor liver or kidney function, doctors will avoid giving medications that can overwork the organs. Giving patient insulin secretagogues is like putting the pancreas into overdrive and will eventually damage the beta cells.

3. Use of Avandia® or Actose®? An experiment in test tubes demonstrated that Avandia might have a protective effect on the beta cell. It will take a few more years to see if it can really protect the patient's beta cells in the pancreas. To me, the reason that they are able to show a protective effect on beta cells is because these medications help to control the blood glucose and lower the A1c. If glucotoxicity is the reason behind beta cell deterioration, then anything that helps with glycemic control will be helpful in preserving the beta cells. This diet is extremely effective in controlling the blood sugar and in the long run I will be able to show that the conclusion of the UKPDS is incorrect. Progressive deterioration of the beta cell is not inevitable.

Fat cells also produce other types of hormones, including Leptin, Interleukin-6, Tumor Necrosis Factor Alpha, Resistin, and Adiponectin, just to name a few. Their role in Type 2 diabetes is not well known yet.

The level of Interleukin-6 level in blood is correlated with the number of adipocytes and insulin resistance. Interleukin-6 induces the production of c-reactive protein (CRP) in the liver, which is an index of inflammation. In turn, the body produces more fibrinogen and platelets, which might increase the chance of blood clot formation and intravascular inflammation[28]. It was concluded that obesity is a risk factor for stroke and heart attack. Normally, Interleukin-6 acts on the central nervous system to decrease the hunger sensation and to increase the metabolic rate. This provides a check and balance on obesity. If you are overeating and produce more adipocytes, the level of Interleukin-6 level also increases and inhibits the appetite and helps you to lose weight. With weight loss and fat loss, the Interlukin-6 level will normalize and will not increase the risk of cardiovascular accident. However, in a patient who develops central nervous system - Interlukin-6 resistance, the body loses its ability to curb the appetite, even with a higher level of Interleukin-6 in systemic circulation. At the same time, the extra amount of Interlukin-6 promotes intravascular inflammation. Remember that it is the adipocytes that produce Interleukin-6. Hence, if you wish to lower the level of Interleukin-6, you have to lose the fat weight. This again demonstrates the principle of treating the cause and not just the symptoms.

Tumor Necrosis Factor Alpha is another cytokine that is found in abundance in obese individuals. Like Interleukin-6, this protein promotes inflammation and insulin resistance, which can be reversed with weight reduction[28-30].

Adiponectin is a hormone produced by the adipose cell. It has a protective effect by improving glucose uptake by the skeletal muscle cells and decreasing gluconeogenesis in the liver cells. Hence, it has a protective effect against diabetes. However, for whatever reason, the production of adiponectin by the adipose cell is blunted in the obese and Type 2 diabetic individuals[31-32]. The level of adiponectin can be increased with the use of thiazolidinediones (Avandia® and Actose®). Hence, this class of drug can enhance insulin sensitivity and inhibit gluconeogenesis[33].

Other medical conditions can also cause glucose intolerance. One example is *Cushing's syndrome*. This condition is due to an excessive amount of blood glucocorticoid hormone, either by intake (taking prednisone for the treatment of autoimmune diseases) or over production (tumor of the adrenal or pituitary gland). Patients with Cushing's syndrome have depleted protein stores as a result of excessive protein catabolism. The skin and subcutaneous tissues are therefore thin, and the muscles are poorly developed. Wounds heal poorly, and minor injuries cause bruises and ecchymoses. Hair growth is inhibited, and the hair is thin and scraggly. Body fat is redistributed in a characteristic way: The extremities are thin, but fat collects in the abdominal wall, face (moon face), and upper back, where it produces a *"buffalo hump."* As the increased subcutaneous fat deposits stretch the thin skin of the abdomen, the subdermal tissues rupture to form prominent reddish-purple striae. These patients can also develop insulin resistance and Type 2 diabetes.

Do not be alarmed if patients gain weight or have an elevated blood glucose level after surgery, trauma or infection. Although the body actually has a heightened metabolic rate, due to other physiological changes, the patient may end up gaining water weight and losing lean muscle mass. Increased levels of catecholamines, glucagon, and glucocorticoids caused insulin suppression, which leads to hyperglycemia. This can also be caused by an increased rate of gluconeogenesis and protein catabolism leading to muscle wasting. Due to the inflammatory reaction, the CRP level increases and the secretion of other acute phase reactants such as Tumor Necrosis Factor Alpha and Interleukin-6 are also elevated. This leads to an increase in heart rate and temperature. Water retention and lower urinary output occurs secondary to augmented vasopressin (ADH) level and mineral corticoid secretion.

Researchers from Johns Hopkins University, Emory University and the University of Wisconsin have discovered a possible link between diabetes and depression. One possible cause is that antidepressants may be causing weight gain. Depressed individuals are also less likely to be compliant with dietary and weight loss recommendations and are more likely to be physically inactive and non-adherent with medications.

Complications of diabetes can be separated into two major categories (Table 9). Microvascular disease is more prominent than macrovascular disease. The risk of both microvascular and macrovascular diseases correlate with the A1c value, which is a function of the postprandial glucose level. For every 1% decrease in A1c, the risk of microvascular complications decrease by 37% and the risk of heart attack decreases by 16%[34].

Table 9. Complications of Diabetes.

Microvascular	Macrovascular
Retinopathy (eye)	Coronary heart disease (heart attack)
Nephropathy (kidney)	Cerebral vascular accident (stroke)
Neuropathy (nerve)	Peripheral vascular disease (circulation)
Erectile dysfunction (impotency)	

Microvascular disease is caused by an over-abundance of glucose in the nerve cells, lens, retinal cells, renal (kidney) cells, blood vessel cells, and pancreatic cells. Remember that insulin is required for glucose to go into the liver, muscle and fat cells. However, insulin is *not* required for glucose to go into the nerve, lens, retinal, renal, blood vessel and pancreatic cells. With diabetes, glucose cannot effectively go into the liver, muscle and fat cells due to an inadequate amount of insulin or due to the presence of insulin resistance. The net effect is an elevated blood glucose, which is transported to the nerve, lens, retinal, renal, blood vessel and pancreatic cells freely. If the glucose in these cells exceeds a certain level, it goes though the *"sorbitol pathway"*, which converts the glucose molecule into sorbitol, and later into fructose. As sorbitol and fructose accumulate inside the cells, they act like sponges and suck water into the cell, leading to swelling, electrolyte imbalance, abnormal cellular function and eventually cell death. This whole process may be reversible if you are able to control your blood glucose before permanent damages are done.

If you able to maintain your blood glucose level in the normal range, then the sorbitol and fructose that are inside the cells will begin to metabolize and convert back into glucose. This leads to normalization of cellular functions as the excessive amount of water leaves the cells. It was found that with every 1% reduction in the glycosylated hemoglobin (A1c) level, there is a 39% reduction in the risk of retinopathy (eye disease) progression. Hence, it is of vital importance to keep the fasting blood glucose level below 5.6 mmol/L and A1c level below 0.060.

Since glucose and water can move in and out of the lens of the eyes freely, independent of the presence or absence of insulin, any dramatic changes in the blood glucose level can alter the shape of the lens and alter the visual acuity. It is not uncommon to find patients with poor diabetic control to improve their glycemic control very quickly on this diet, and may therefore complain of blurry vision. As mentioned before, the doctor just has to reassure the patients that this is a normal phenomenon and that will improve with time once the blood glucose level is stabilized.

The relationship between diabetes and macrovascular disease is not as clear-cut. We know that the risk of heart attack and stroke increases with diabetes. However, we do not know if high blood glucose itself is an independent factor for these events, or if it is worsening the underlying risk factors for cardiovascular disease. For example, insulin resistance is known to cause high blood pressure, increase serum cholesterol and triglycerides levels, and worsening of arteriosclerosis.

The type of patient that we treat in our clinic is the obese, Type 2 diabetic with poor glycemic (blood glucose) control. The million-dollar question is "which diet is best for this type of patient who needs to lose weight and get the blood glucose into the normal range?" Most patients have taken diabetic clinic classes and received dietary counseling from their dieticians. The recommendation given to them is very similar to that of the Canada Food Guide for Health Eating: Eat "healthy" with plenty of fresh fruits and vegetables, but limit the protein and fat intake. The following meal plans are copied from the *Canadian Diabetic Association* website. It was developed by the Implementation Subcommittee of the National Nutrition Committee in 1999 to help health care professionals to counsel their diabetic patients.

Sample Meal Plans
(Canadian Diabetic Association)

For Small Appetites

Breakfast:

Cereal (½ cup, 125 ml)
Toast (1 slice)
1 orange
Milk (1 cup, 250 ml)
Peanut butter (1 tbsp, 15 ml)
Tea or coffee

Lunch:

1 Sandwich
- 2 slices of whole grain bread or 6" pita
- meat, chicken or fish (2 oz, 60 g)
- margarine or mayonnaise (1 tsp., 5 ml)
Carrot sticks, 10 small
Fruit yogurt (½ cup, 125 ml)
Tea or coffee

Dinner:

Potato (1 medium) or rice (1/3 cup, 150 ml)
Vegetables
Margarine or butter (1 tsp., 5 ml)
Lean meat, chicken, or fish (2 oz, 60 g)
¼ cantaloupe
Milk (1 cup, 250 ml)
Tea or coffee
Evening snack:
Low fat cheese (1 oz, 30 g)
Soda crackers (6)

For Big Appetites

Breakfast:

Cereal (½ cup, 125 ml)
Toast (2 slices) or 1 small bagel
1 Orange
Milk (1 cup, 250 ml)
Peanut butter (2 tbsp., 30 ml)
Tea or coffee

Lunch:

Soup (1 cup, 250 ml)
Sandwich
- 2 slices whole grain bread or 6" pita
- lean meat, chicken, or fish (3 oz, 90 g)
- tomato slices
- margarine or mayonnaise (1tsp, 5 ml)
Carrot sticks, 10 small
Fruit yogurt (½ cup, 125 ml)
Tea or coffee

Afternoon snack:

1 medium apple or banana

Dinner:

1 large potato or cooked noodles (1½ cup, 375 ml)
Vegetables
Margarine or butter (1 tsp., 5 ml)
Green salad with lemon juice
Lean meat, chicken or fish (4 oz, 120 g)
1 Pear
Milk (1 cup, 250 ml)
Tea or coffee
Evening snack:
Low fat cheese (2 oz, 60 g)
Melba toast (4)
Milk (1 cup, 250 ml)

This is a typical low-protein-low-fat-high-carbohydrate diet that Health Canada has been promoting. How are patients able to attain glycemic control with this amount of sugar and starch in their diet? In the past, the Canada Food Guide and the Canadian Diabetic Association (CDA) have not been concerned with sugar intake. They believe that it is the total calorie rather than carbohydrate intake that cause obesity. In the CDA web site, www.diabetes.ca, you can find a recipe for a chocolate chip cookie bar! Recently the CDA lowered the daily carbohydrate intake to about 200 grams and stressed the importance of eating complex carbohydrates, i.e. with low glycemic indexes (GI). However, the CDA did not take glycemic load (GL) into consideration. Studies have found that it is not the type of carbohydrate you eat but the total amount of carbohydrates that you consumed that elevates blood glucose and A1c. If you follow a diet prescribed to you that is high in carbohydrates, your post meal blood glucose might elevate. Unless you do a lot of cardiovascular exercises daily and take medications to lower the blood glucose, your diabetes will be difficult to control. For the obese diabetic patient, is this too much to ask? Is it really practical in the real world? If you eat sugar and starch, and then inject insulin to lower the blood glucose, you are just moving the blood glucose from the blood stream into the adipocytes, which just lead to more fat formation and thus weight gain. The WHO proposed that for diabetic patients, their BMI should be kept around 21 to 23, but how can the obese diabetic patient lose weight by eating sugar? Why are we feeding sugar to poorly controlled diabetic patients? Why are we telling patients to eat sugar and then prescribing them pills or injections to lower their blood glucose? Why do we have to eat sugar at all? Is a "no" glycemic index diet better than a low glycemic index diet? This is strictly my own viewpoint and is totally different from mainstream diabetic teaching. It is not easy to change old schools of thought without having results from randomised double blind studies using thousands of obese diabetic patients. I do not have the resources to do this kind of study.

Healthy Eating ≠ Weight Reduction

Healthy Eating ≠ Sugar Control

The Canada Food Guide for Healthy Eating recommends that 55% of your daily calorie intake should be coming from carbohydrates. In the 80's, Canadian used to have only 48% of the daily calories intake come from carbohydrates. Canadians are getting fatter and more diagnoses of Type 2 (adult onset) diabetes. There is no scientific evidence that we need to eat 300 grams of carbohydrates per day (as recommended by the food guide in the past). It is totally arbitrary. Keep in mind that I do not disagree that the Canada Food Guide is healthy for the average Canadian. What I wish to point out to the reader is that the recommendations from the food guide are not useful in treating obesity or chronic disease.

With a diet that is low in sugar and starch, your daily insulin requirement will be less. Hence you will be taking less medication and/or insulin leading to weight loss and better blood glucose control. Our diet builds on this principle and is very effective in controlling the blood glucose. It was found that glucose produced from eating protein does not end up in the blood stream and that eating protein does not affect the blood glucose level. Another upside of eating protein is that it helps to build muscle (especially with muscle building exercises), which increases the ability to dispose of blood glucose (glucose clearance). Substitution of dietary protein for carbohydrate improves overall glucose control without increasing the risk of heart disease[34-35].

There are variations of Type 2 diabetes that should be mentioned here to physicians and other health care professionals who take care of diabetic patients. One subgroup of Type 2 diabetic patients presents with complications found in Type 1 diabetic patients: Diabetic ketoacidosis, polydipsia (frequent drinking due to increase in thirst), polyurea (frequent urination) and weight loss, just like what a Type 1 diabetic would. However, there are a few features that do not quit fit the Type 1 diabetic picture. These patients are usually in their forties (versus childhood onset), obese or overweight, and the disease usually goes into remission spontaneously (showing normal C-peptide levels). Some patients in this subgroup do eventually require some form of anti-diabetic treatment. One key feature that separates this subgroup of Type 2 diabetic patients from the Type 1 diabetic patients is the absence of antibodies toward insulin, islet cell and glutamic acid decarboxylase (GAB). Do not assume that all patients who have been hospitalized for severe hyperglycemia and ketoacidosis are Type 1 diabetics and require insulin injections for life.

Another Type 2 diabetic subgroup presents with a typical Type 2 diabetic history and laboratory examinations. However, this group of patients eventually develops antibodies towards GAB, and low or negative insulin and C-peptide levels. This subgroup of patients will require daily insulin injections.

Hypertension, Dyslipidemia and Coronary Heart Disease

High blood pressure for the general population is defined as mean systolic blood pressure > 140 mm Hg, or mean diastolic blood pressure > 90 mm Hg, or currently taking anti-hypertensive medication. However, the normal blood pressure for diabetic and/or kidney patients should be lowered to 130/80. The target value is further lowered to 125/75 if there is protein in the urine. The prevalence of high blood pressure in adults with BMI > 30 is 38.4 percent for men and 32.2 percent for women, respectively, compared with 18.2 percent for men and 16.5 percent for women with BMI < 25, a relative risk of 2.1 and 1.9 for men and women, respectively.

The direct and independent association between blood pressure and BMI or weight has been shown in numerous studies. One study reported that a 10 kg (22 lb.) rise in body weight is associated with 3.0 mm Hg higher systolic and 2.3 mm Hg higher diastolic blood pressure. These differences in blood pressure translate into an estimated 12 percent increased risk for coronary heart disease, and 24 percent increased risk for stroke.

Obesity and hypertension are co-morbid risk factors for the development of cardiovascular disease and stroke (Table 10). The pathophysiology underlying the development of hypertension associated with obesity includes sodium retention and an associated increase in vascular resistance, blood volume, and cardiac output. These are related to a combination of increased sympathetic nervous system tone, alterations of the renin-angiotensin system (adipocytes secrete angiotensinogen), and insulin resistance. Essential hypertension now also is considered to be an insulin-resistant state, based on epidemiological, clinical and experimental studies. Insulin can increase sympathetic nervous system activity by facilitating glucose uptake in neurons within the hypothalamus. Subsequently this induces hypertension by causing vasoconstriction and renal sodium retention[36]. People with insulin resistance are more likely to have salt-sensitive hypertension[37]. Hence patients with metabolic syndrome are very sensitive to sodium in their diet. A small increase of in the sodium in the diet can produce a sharp rise in blood pressure. The net effect will be congestive heart failure. Randeree HA et al found that systolic blood pressure rose by about 16 mm Hg and diastolic blood pressure rose by about 8 mm Hg over 3 months of follow-up in people with Type 2 diabetes after initiation of insulin[38]. In another study, Tedde R et al found a fall in blood pressure in hypertensive women with Type 2 diabetes after a reduction in their insulin dose[39].

It is a well known fact that obese patients have increased circulating free fatty acids, which increases glucose production and induces hyperinsulinemia. It also increases the circulating Very Low Density Lipoprotein (VLDL) and decreases the High Density Lipoprotein (HDL) and increases the small dense Low Density Lipoprotein (LDL). Increased free fatty acid blocks the uptake of glucose by muscle and the extra glucose will be transformed into fat and thus increases in the formation of fat in the muscle. An increase in insulin causes an elevation of BP by increasing sodium retention. An increase in the number of adipocytes increases the production of Tumor Necrosis Factor Alpha and Intraleukin-6, which increases the production of CRP by the liver, decreases adiponectin and decreases insulin sensitivity. All these are potential mechanisms of the metabolic syndrome (see chapter 5).

Table 10. Effect of Obesity on the Cardiovascular System.	
1.	Increase Heart Rate (Decrease Parasympathetic Tone)
2.	Increase Cardiac Output (Increase Extracellular Volume)
3.	Increase Size of Heart Muscle (Cardiac Hypertrophy)
4.	Increase Blood Pressure (Increase Renal Sodium Reabsorption)
5.	Increase Sympathetic Tone
6.	Increase Renin - Angiotensin Production

Most obese patients will have abnormal lipid profiles: a low level of HDL (cholesterol), a high level of LDL (bad cholesterol), and elevated VLDL (triglycerides). Triglycerides and VLDL are related to insulin resistance and hyperinsulinemia. With insulin resistance, the liver produces an excess amount of triglycerides. Remember that 80% of blood cholesterol is produced in vivo (by you) and is controlled by genetic factors. If it is due to genetic factors, even the best diet and weight loss program may not be able to return the LDL cholesterol to the normal value. However, this does not mean that we are not going to try. Conversely, eating food that is higher in good fat may not elevate the blood cholesterol. Of all the food ingredients, it was found that eating a diet that is high in saturated fat and carbohydrates are the real culprit for blood cholesterol elevation.

Your blood lipid profiles (total cholesterol, LDL, HDL, and triglycerides) measure lipids that you have ingested and lipids that you have produced from your liver. Hence when your blood test result comes back abnormal, you do not know if it is high because you have eaten too much fat and/or carbohydrate, and/or your liver is making too much cholesterol.

Table 11. Lipoprotein Electrophoresis Patterns.

Type	Synonyms	Appearance of Serum	Changes in Lipid	Treatment Principle
I (rare)	Familial (Essential) Hypertrigly-ceridemia	Cream layer on top, clear below	Cholesterol ⇑ Triglycerides ⇑	Restrict fat intake
IIa (common)	Familial (Essential) hyper-cholesterolemia	Clear	Cholesterol ⇑ Triglycerides Normal	Medication, weight control
IIb	Mixed Hyper-lipoproteinemia (Overindulgence Hyperlipemia)	Slightly turbid	Cholesterol ⇑ Triglycerides ⇑	Diet, may need medication
III (less common)	Familial Hyperlipemia	Turbid with faint cream layer	Cholesterol ⇑ Triglycerides ⇑	Diet and medication
IV (most common)	Carbohydrate-induced Hyperlipemia	Turbid without cream layer	Cholesterol ⇑ Triglycerides ⇑	Weight reduction, low-carb and limit alcohol intake
V (un-common)	Mixed Type I and Type IV	Cream layer on top, turbid below	Cholesterol ⇑ or Normal, Triglycerides ⇑	Diet and medication

If you do not eat fat at all, and you have a strong family history of high cholesterol, you probably have a bad gene that causes you to produce cholesterol in the liver. This is called *Essential Familial Hypercholesterolemia* (Type IIa). The blood test will show high concentrations of cholesterol and normal amount of triglycerides (Table 11). Dietary manipulation will probably not be successful in the treatment of this type of patient. They should be treated with medications. Doing a blood test called *Lipoprotein electrophoresis* may help you identify this group of patients. Once you label the patient as having Familial Hypercholesterolemia, you are committing the patient to take medication for life (after you rule out other metabolic causes).

By far, the most common cause of abnormal lipid profiles is due to the over consumption of carbohydrates. This is also known as *Carbohydrate-induced Hyperlipemia* (Type IV). The blood test will indicate a normal or high cholesterol level and high triglycerides level. The treatment of this kind of hyperlipemia is through weight reduction and lowering the carbohydrate and alcohol consumption.

Essential or Familial Hypertriglyceridemia (Type I) is rare.

Mixed Hyperlipoproteinemia (Type IIb) is from long-term overindulgence of fat. Both cholesterol and triglycerides are high in the blood test. Diet alone is probably adequate but may need reinforcement with medication.

Product monograms of Lipitor® and Crestor®, two commonly used cholesterol lowering medications, state that "Before instituting therapy, an attempt should be made to control hypercholesterolemia with appropriate diet, exercises, weight reduction in overweight patients, and to treat other underlying medical problems (poorly controlled diabetes, hypothyroidism, nephrotic syndrome, dysproteinemias, obstructive liver disease, and alcoholism) and associated cardiovascular risk factors." This is because many other medical problems can cause hyperlipoproteinemia (Table 12).

Table 12. Hyperlipoproteinemia Secondary to or Associated with Specific Disorders.

Type	Disorders
I	Uncontrolled diabetes, Pancreatitis, Acute alcoholism, Hypothyroidism, Hyperestrogenemia
II	Diet high in saturated fat or cholesterol, Hypothyroidism, Obstructive hepatic disease, Hypoproteinemia, Multiple myeloma, Macroglobinemia, Hypercalcemia, Acute porphyria
III	Hypothyroidism, Dysglobulinemias, Hepatic disease, Diabetes
IV	Diabetes, Pancreatitis, Acute Alcoholism, Glycogen storage disease, Hypothyroidism, Nephrotic syndrome, Hyperglobulinemia, Pregnancy, Gout
V	Diabetes, Acute Alcoholism, Chronic Pancreatitis

An increase in blood glucose level as in a poorly controlled diabetic patient triggers insulin secretion from the pancreas. Insulin increases the HMR-CoA reductase activity, which leads to an increase in the production of cholesterol. The most commonly used group of medication to lower patient's LDL level is called "statins". It works by inhibiting the activity of the HMR-CoA reductase. If this patient can control his blood glucose level, there will be no need for the pancreas to secret extra amount of insulin and the HMR-CoA reductase will remain calm. Realistically, it is the sugar and starch in the diet that raises the blood glucose. If the patient avoids eating sugar and starch, the blood glucose will not go up and the production of the LDL will also decrease. Figure 6 demonstrates that LDL and triglycerides synthesis is in direct proportion to the blood glucose level.

Figure 6. Production of Triglycerides and Cholesterol form Glucose.

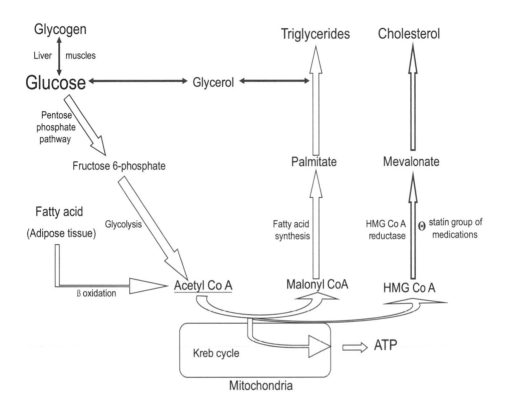

In 2003, the "normal values" of cholesterol, LDL, and HDL have been replaced by "target levels", depending on your risk category of coronary artery disease (Table 13). For example, if you belong to the high-risk category (Type 2 diabetic, and a patient who has pre-existing cardiovascular disease), your risk of having coronary artery disease in the next 10 years is more than 20%. Then, in order to avoid a heart attack, your target LDL cholesterol level should be less than 2.5 mmol/L, and your Total to HDL cholesterol ratio should be below 4.0.

Table 13. Target Cholesterol Levels According to Risk Category.

Risk Category	10-Year Risk of Coronary Heart Disease	Target LDL Cholesterols (mmol/L)	Target Total: HDL Ratio
High	20%	< 2.5	< 4.0
Moderate	10-19%	3.5	< 5.0
Low	< 10%	< 4.5	< 6.0

To figure out which risk category you belong to, answer the questions on Table 14. It is based on your age, gender, cholesterol, blood pressure, smoking, and family history.

Table 14. Estimate the 10-year Risk of Coronary Events in Patient without Diabetes or Cardiovascular Disease.

Look up the number of points corresponding to your age and gender

Age	Male	Female
20 - 34	-9	-7
35 - 39	-4	-3
40 - 44	0	0
45 - 49	3	3
50 - 54	6	6
55 - 59	8	8
60 - 64	10	10
65 - 69	11	12
70 - 74	12	14
75 - 79	13	16

Total Cholesterol (mmol/L)

Look up the number of points corresponding to your age and total cholesterol (mmol/l) level

Age	20 - 39 Male	20 - 39 Female	40 - 49 Male	40 - 49 Female	50 - 59 Male	50 - 59 Female	60 - 69 Male	60 - 69 Female	70 - 79 Male	70 - 79 Female
< 4.1	0	0	0	0	0	0	0	0	0	0
4.1 - 5.1	4	4	3	3	2	2	1	1	0	1
5.2 - 6.1	7	8	5	6	3	4	7	7	0	1
6.2 - 7.2	9	11	6	8	4	5	2	3	1	2
> 7.3	11	13	8	10	5	7	3	4	1	2

Skip this part if you are a non-smoker. Look up the number of points corresponding to your age if you smoke

Smoker

	8	9	5	7	3	4	1	2	1	1

Look up the number of points corresponding to your age and HDL cholesterol (mmol/l) level

HDL (mmol/L)

	Male	Female
> 1.6	-1	-1
1.3 - 1.5	0	0
1.0 - 1.2	1	1
< 1.0	2	2

Look up the number of points corresponding to your systolic blood pressure (mmHg)

Systolic Blood Pressure (mmHg)

	Untreated Male	Untreated Female	Treated Male	Treated Female
> 120	0	0	0	0
120 - 129	0	1	1	3
130 - 139	1	2	2	4
140 - 159	1	3	2	5
< 160	2	4	3	6

Add up all the points and estimate your 10-year risk below:																		
Males																		
Points total:	<0	0	1	2	3	4	5	6	7	8	9	10	11	12	13	14	15	16	>17
10 year risk %	<1	1	1	1	1	1	2	2	3	4	5	6	8	10	12	16	20	25	>30
Females																		
Points total:	<9	9	10	11	12	13	14	15	16	17	18	19	20	21	22	23	24	>25
10 year risk %	<1	1	1	1	1	2	2	3	4	5	6	8	11	14	17	22	27	>30

Using data from one of my patients as an example, patient KC is a 48 year old male (3 points). His total cholesterol is 6.3 mmol/L (6 points), non-smoker (0 point), HDL is 1.1 mmol/L (1 point), and untreated systolic blood pressure is 143 mmHg (1 point). He yields a total of 11 points. Hence, his 10-year risk is 8% and puts him in the "low risk" category. His LDL cholesterol target will be any level <4.5 and the Total to HDL cholesterol ratio target will be anything <6.0.

Here is another example: Mrs. MG is 63 years old (10 points) and has a total cholesterol value of 6.0 mmol/L (2 points). She smokes (2 points) and her HDL cholesterol is 0.8 mmol/L (2 points). While on antihypertensive medications, her systolic blood pressure is 145 mmHg (5 points). She scores a total of 21 points which puts her in the "moderate risk" category (10-year risk is 14 %). Her target for LDL cholesterol will be <3.5 mmol/L with a ratio of <5.0.

Recent recommendations suggest that if you have a first degree relative that has cardiovascular disease or diabetes, you should double your 10-year risk. If Mr. KC has a father suffering from diabetes, then he should double his 10-year risk from 8% to 16% putting him in the "moderate risk" category instead.

We are told that a high level of the good HDL cholesterol, can balance out the bad LDL cholesterol. Recent trial shows that LDL is a risk factor for developing coronary heart disease regardless of your HDL levels. Some cardiologists suggest that the lower the LDL level the better.

Doctors measure the LDL level because they want to assess the risk of developing atherogenic plaque. However, LDL is not the only type of fat that causes plaque formation. Very Low Density Lipoprotein (VLDL), Intermediate Density Lipoprotein, and lipoprotein-a are all capable of produce plaque. Each of these atherogenic fat molecules contains one molecule of Apo-lipoprotein B. Hence the measurement of the serum Apo-lipoprotein B level gives you a better assessment of cardiovascular risk than measuring the LDL level alone. Another benefit of measuring Apo-lipoprotein B over LDL is that fasting sample is not necessary.

Do not confuse lipoprotein-a with Apolipoprotein-A1. Apolipoprotein A1 is produced by the liver and its function is to bind cholesterol and phospholipids. The higher the Apolipoprotein-A1 level, the higher the serum HDL level. Hence, lipoprotein-a is bad and Apolipoprotein-A1 is good. A class of medication called fibrates increases the serum HDL level by activating the peroxisome proliferator-activated receptor alpha (PPARα) and subsequently increases the Apolipoprotein-A1 level. Peroxisome proliferator-activated receptor gamma (PPARγ) is another nuclear receptor activator that is responsible for insulin sensitivity and glucose metabolism. PPARγ can be activated by Actose® and Avandia®.

Hypertriglyceridemia means elevated concentration of fat in the blood stream. It is considered atherogenic (causes thickening and hardening of artery), which can lead to occlusion or thrombosis of the artery. Stroke or heart attack may follow. Hypertriglyceridemia can be caused by genetic and/or acquired factors (Tables 11 and 12). Drugs that elevate the serum triglycerides level include beta blockers, diuretics, hormone replacement therapy, tamoxifen and prednisone. Serum triglycerides level and HDL level are inversely proportional to each other. If the triglycerides level is high, the HDL level will be low. Achievement of the target HDL level usually entails modification of the triglycerides level when elevated[40].

Lipoprotein lipase is an important enzyme that is responsible for the removal of triglycerides from the blood stream. This enzyme is produced in the adipocytes and migrates to the endothelial cell of the capillaries. The production of lipoprotein lipase is related to the amount of circulating insulin. In the obese insulin resistant subject, the production of lipoprotein lipase is impaired, which leads to a decrease in the clearance of serum triglycerides and an increase in the risk of atherogenic plaque formation.

In a review article in the New England Journal of Medicine, it concluded that one can lower the cardiovascular risk by increasing the HDL cholesterol level. Commonly used drugs that can elevate the HDL cholesterol level are niacin (20-30%), fibrates (10-25%), and statins (2-15%). Lifestyle modifications such as exercise, weight loss and moderate alcohol consumption are also effective in raising the HDL cholesterol level. Weight loss achieved through exercise is more effective at raising HDL levels than dieting. Genetic disorders characterized by a low HDL concentration are rare and include mutations in apolipoprotein A-1, the major protein component of HDL[41]. On the other hand, a diet high in carbohydrates will lower the level of HDL cholesterol through raising the triglycerides level.

Fructose increases triglycerides formation, even more so than glucose or sucrose[42]. A high fructose diet (fruit and juice) overwhelms the liver glycogenesis and increases fatty acid synthesis leading to an increase in triglycerides after a meal. The effect is worse if the subject is already has a high serum triglycerides and suffering from insulin resistance. Fructose is naturally present in honey and fruit or by isomerization of glucose from corn in the form of high-fructose corn syrup that is used in abundance in soft drinks.

As discussed earlier, adipocytes secrete an adipokine called Interleukin-6 that leads to an increase of the circulating C - reactive protein (CRP). CRP is associated with chronic inflammation (rheumatoid arthritis) and acute coronary syndrome (death of heart muscle with angina)[43]. Normally, Interleukin-6 acts on the central nervous system to decrease the hunger sensation and increases metabolic rate. This provides a check and balance on obesity. If you are overeating and produce more adipocytes, the level of Interleukin-6 level also increases and inhibits the appetite and helps one to lose weight. With weight loss and fat loss, the Interlukin-6 level will normalize and will not increase the risk of a cardiovascular accident. However, in patient who develops central nervous system - Interleukin-6 resistance the body loses its ability to curb the appetite, even with high level of Interleukin-6 level in systemic circulation. The patient will not be able to curb the appetite. At the same time, the extra amount of Interleukin-6 promotes intravascular inflammation. Remember, it is the adipocytes that produce Interleukin-6. Hence if you want to lower the level of circulating Interlukin-6, you have to lose fat weight. This again demonstrates the principle of treating cause and not the symptom.

CRP are produced mainly form the liver and partially from the cardiac smooth muscles. Elevated CRP levels in the blood carry a negative effect for coronary heart disease. The plaques inside the arteries of patients with high CRP levels are found to be unstable and more prone to rupture. CRP levels can be lowered with cessation of smoking, weight reduction, increase in physical activity or taking statins and/or fibrates medications. Fish oil and flaxseed oil may be useful also. Decrease in the CPR level can translate into lowering the risk of heart attack, independent of the LDL level.

Tumor Necrosis Factor Alpha is another adipokine that found in abundance in obese individuals. Like Interleukin-6, this protein promotes inflammation and insulin resistance.

Obese patients carry a ten-fold increase in sudden cardiac death because of an increase risk of arrhythmia. The QT interval on the ECG may be prolonged in the obese patient and indicates a higher risk of sudden death. The QT interval is measured from the beginning of the Q wave to the end of the T wave. A normal QT interval is 0.33 to 0.45 seconds. Do a baseline ECG to check for arrhythmias and the QT interval. It was suggested that one should repeat the ECG with every 50 pounds of weight loss.

A high percentage of obese patients also have hyperinsulinemia. The insulin stimulates the kidneys to retain salt and water by releasing other hormones such as cortisol and aldosterone[37-38]. Insulin also promotes the loss of magnesium through the urine. A low magnesium level has been shown to elevate blood pressure. Hence, we recommend that hypertensive patients on this diet program take a magnesium supplement. Insulin promotes the growth of smooth muscle cells in the wall of the arteries and leads to narrowing of the lumen of the arteries. Another way to cause artery damage is through the increase in plaque formation. Plasminogen Activator Inhibitor, a factor that inhibits blood clots form dissolving, is increased in obese patients. The fibrinogen level in blood is an independent risk factor in coronary heart disease that is not related to cholesterol. The higher the fibrinogen level, the higher the risk of thrombosis (blood clotting inside the coronary artery) and heart attack. Your doctor may wish to measure the serum fibrinogen level to assess the risk of developing coronary heart disease. However, there is no effective means of lowering the fibrinogen level.

Non-drug approaches are front and center in the 2004 guidelines for the management of hypertension. The guidelines put the emphasis on lifestyle changes and prevention.

Treatment options of essential hypertension and dyslipidemia related to obesity are:

1. Weight loss, which is associated with a reduction in vascular resistance and total blood volume and cardiac output, improvement in insulin resistance and ventricular function, a reduction in sympathetic tone, and suppression of the activity of the renin-angiotensin aldosterone system.

2. Increased physical activity. Cardiopulmonary exercise such as walking, jogging, cycling or swimming for 30 to 45 minutes, three to five times per week

3. Decrease sodium intake

4. Stop smoking

5. Stress management. Both psychological and physical stress (illness, chronic pain, or lack of sleep to name a few) increases the secretion of adrenaline and causes high blood pressure.

6. Diet high in fiber and low in saturated fat

7. Limit alcohol to less than two drinks per day

8. Medications. Angiotensin Converting Enzyme (ACE) inhibitors (Monopril®, Vasotec®, Coversyl®, Altace®, Zestril®, Prinivil®, Capoten®, Marvik®, etc) suppress the renin-angiotensin system, which is usually over reactive in obese patients. Some of their side effects are cough, hyperkalemia (high serum potassium level) and angioedema (allergic reaction). Angiotensin Receptor Blockers (Diovan®, Avapro®, Micardis®, Cozaar®, Atacand®, etc) have a smaller chance of cough and angioedema. The newest class of antihypertensive is called renin inhibitor (Rasilez®). The older class of antihypertensive such as alpha blockers, beta blockers, calcium channel blockers and diuretics are all useful to lower the blood

pressure. However, they may not be suitable in some situations. Let your doctor or specialist recommend them for you. Use of statin medications (Lipitor®, Crestor®, Zocor®, Pravachol®, etc.) have been shown to reduce the risk of coronary events in patients with a high cholesterol level. What is interesting is that for people with normal cholesterol level but are of high risk (previous heart attack, hypertension or diabetes), a low dose statin medication taken daily reduces the chance of acute heart attack. This protective effect may be due to the stabilization effect of statin medications on the atherosclerotic plaque (reduced inflammation, improved endothelial function, reduced plaque lipid and oxidized LDL content, and increased antithrombotic and pro-fibrinolytic activity). A patient who takes statin medication has a dose-related reduction in the CRP level. The more aggressive the dose of statin medication, the higher of percentage of CRP reduction. Drugs of choice for hypertriglyceridemia are nicotinic acid and fibrates (Lipidil®). Lipidil® may also raise the HDL level, which is cardio-protective. It may be used in conjunction with other statin-type medications. However, the risk of side effects is elevated when they are used together. Routine laboratory monitoring of the liver function and muscle damage is necessary. The addition of fiber supplementation to statin medication can help to lower the cholesterol further. Ezetrol® is a class of medication called cholesterol absorption inhibitor. It blocks the reabsorption of cholesterol from the bile secreted from the gall bladder. It can be used on its own or in combination with a statin type medication. Laboratory testing is also required. Niacin is one of the B vitamins and is actually more effective in elevating the HDL level than prescription medications (see chapter 14). Niacin reduces the clearance of HDL, hence increasing the circulating HDL level.

Case # 4. Mrs. ED is a 60 year old retired nurse who is suffering from hypertension, chronic indigestion and high serum triglycerides. Her weight was 183 pounds, she is five foot three inches, with a BMI of 32.5 and a 44% total body fat. Her usual medications were 80 mg of

Diovan®, 20 mg of Losec® and 12.5 mg of hydrochlorothiazide per day. Upon reviewing her blood work report that was done before dieting, her fasting blood glucose was elevated at 6.9 mmol/L. This indicates impaired fasting glucose. Her serum triglycerides were also high. Hydrochlorothiazide is not a good choice for her because it can worsen the blood glucose and lipid profile. Three months into the diet, all three medications were discontinued since there was no need for them. Her weight was 150 pounds, and her percent body fat dropped to 35%. Her blood work showed a normal level of fasting glucose (4.4 mmol/L) and triglycerides (0.77 mmol/L). On the fifth month, without any medication, her blood pressure was still 118/70. The percent body fat was 31% and her weight was 141 pounds. She was given the maintenance diet.

Obesity and Cancer

Obesity is linked to breast, uterine, prostate, kidney, colon, esophageal, and pancreatic cancer. Obesity induces tumor growth by:

1. Increasing the production of hormones by the adipose tissue that binds to tumor cells and promotes their growth. For example, estrogen is produced by the adipose tissue and stimulates breast cancer growth and metastasis. Men with prostate cancer who consume higher amounts of fat demonstrate faster tumor growth. In contrast, eating a protein rich diet may slow down tumor growth.

2. Decreasing hormone-binding globulin level and increasing the free circulating hormone level.

3. Increasing oxidant stress and promoting cell proliferation and DNA damage. For example, androgens increase oxidant stress in the prostate cancer cells.

4. Adipose tissue produces *cytokines* that stimulate the production of steroid hormones in cancer cells.

Obese patients should have routine mammography, colonoscopy and serum prosthetic specific antigen (PSA) done yearly. Any obese female patients with abnormal virginal bleeding should have a pelvic ultrasound and/or endometrial biopsy. Hematurea and/or unexplained hypertension require a renal ultrasound and/or cystoscopy. Epigastric pain requires upper GI and abdominal ultrasound and/or CT scan.

The use of antioxidants in cancer prevention is still controversial. Supplementation with vitamins and antioxidants in the recommended dosage range will never hurt. No one knows if weight reduction decreases the risk of cancer. Most studies compare obese subjects with normal weight subjects. There is no study that compares the cancer risk pre and post weight loss. One thing is for sure, obesity increases your risk of the cancers mentioned above. Pay attention to your weight if there is a family history of any of the cancers mentioned above.

Autoimmune Disease

Obese people are more prone to developing autoimmune diseases such as celiac disease, thyroiditis and Grave's disease, autoimmune hepatitis, myasthenia gravis, rheumatoid arthritis, multiple sclerosis, lupus, ulcerative colitis and Crohn's disease, psoriasis, etc. The biogenetic cause is still unknown.

Grain products were introduced for human consumption about 10 thousand years ago. Before this time, men were mainly relying on animal products. Due to its relatively recent introduction, our species has not fully adapted physiologically to its digestion and metabolism.

Grain contains many metabolic components commonly categorized as anti-nutrients. Anti-nutrients are chemical compounds naturally occurring in most food products but are found in much higher concentrations in grain products. Anti-nutrients block the absorption of nutrients in our diet. For example, phytic acid in grain products forms insoluble complexes with calcium, zinc, iron and copper[44]. Trypsin inhibitors, tennins, and lectins are some other examples of anti-nutrients. Recent scientific study has linked these anti-nutrients to a number of diseases, which include allergen based disorders, pancreatic hypertrophy and disruption of the gut cell wall tight junctions (thus exposing the systemic circulation to food allergens). When the body develops an allergic reaction to these anti-nutrients, it causes a cross-reaction to our own body, leading to autoimmune diseases.

CRP is a protein produced in the liver in response to inflammatory conditions such as rheumatoid arthritis. The blood level of CRP coincides with the severity of the disease. A high level of CRP indicates that there is a flare up of the arthritis. When treated with medications, the CRP level comes down and the pain subsides. Another way to decrease the CRP level is by weight reduction. The normal value of CRP is higher in people with a higher body mass index. The CRP level is often elevated in patients with metabolic syndrome (Chapter 5).

Acne and Other Skin Disorders

Acne is a multifactorial disease. A recent study suggested that a diet rich in refined carbohydrates (junk foods) boosts insulin and subsequently stimulate sebaceous secretion and leads to clogged pores, bacterial growth and acne vulgaris.

A landmark study done by Dr. Gerd Plewig 40 years ago looking at the relationship between acne and chocolate consumption concluded that eating chocolate does not cause acne. Medical doctors have been giving their patients the same message ever since. However, patients and doctors alike reported that their acne was made worse with the ingestion of junk foods, especially chips and soda. When one looks back to the study done by Dr. Plewig, the chocolate group and the placebo group actually consume the same amount of carbohydrates. If carbohydrates, especially sugar, are the real cause of acne, then it is natural that Dr. Plewig found no difference between both groups in the amount of acne production. However, this is only an observation and more research is needed. If junk foods do not cause acne, it sure can aggravate it.

Obesity and insulin resistance can cause acne vulgaris. Obese female patients usually have an imbalance of hormones. The male hormone testosterone is excessively produced by the ovaries and adipocytes because of insulin resistance, which causes an increase in insulin secretion, and leads to an increase in sebaceous secretion from the pores. This group of female patients will also show features of hirsutism (increase in facial hair).

A skin condition known as *Acanthosis nigricans* can be found in patients with severe insulin resistance, Type 2 diabetes, polycystic ovary syndrome or gastrointestinal cancer. Patients with Acanthosis nigricans usually have pigmented plaques on the axillae, elbow crease, nape of the neck and other skin folds. Multiple skin tags may also be present.

Stretch marks (striae) are caused by the tearing of the dermis of the skin when rapid growth occurs such as during pregnancy, puberty and rapid weight gain. The color of the striae starts out as red or purple. The intensity of the color may fade with time but will never disappear completely. No cream or laser treatment can provide complete resolution of the striae. It is of pure cosmetic reasons to treat striae, as they do not pose any health threat.

Other skin conditions such as male pattern hair loss in pre-menopausal females, stasis dermatitis in the lower limbs, psoriasis, keratosis pilaris, dry skin, varicose vein, lymphedema, plantar hyperkeratosis (thickening of skin at the sole of the feet) and folliculitis are all associated with obesity.

Water Retention

Many obese patients have swollen legs. This can be due to excessive water retention, renal diseases, hormonal imbalance, premenstrual symptoms, varicose veins, venous stasis, thrombophebitis, poor nutritional state, liver disease, deep vein thrombosis, congestive heart failure, weather, and/or medications. The physician needs to obtain a thorough medical and familial history taking and perform a thorough examination to determine the cause of the swelling.

There are a few reasons that obese patients retain water (e.g. increase sympathetic activity, activation of the renin-angiotensin system, and hyperinsulinemia). The final pathway of all these mechanisms is the retention of sodium by the kidney. This diet, through lowering of the insulin level, utilization of glycogen, and the production of ketone bodies, is effective in getting rid of some of the peripheral edema.

Swelling of the lower extremity often results in a reddish rash to the skin know as *stasis dermatitis*. Treatment involves decreasing the pressure on the skin through the removal of the edema. The doctors usually prescribe compression stockings, limb elevation, and/or a diuretic(s). However, diuretic has many side effects such as worsening of glycemic and lipid control, weight gain (rather than weight lost), gout, orthostatic hypotension, and electrolyte imbalance (lower your sodium and potassium). It is very important for this type of patient to stay on a low sodium diet, even if they are taking diuretic, unless the serum sodium level is low. Diuretics act by causing sodium to be excreted in the urine, thus drawing water along with it. If you take salt (sodium chloride) in your diet, you are defeating the purpose of taking diuretic. You have just replaces the sodium you excreted into the urine when you take diuretic. Water will be retained in your body. The best way to get rid of water retention is to treat the cause of the retention.

There are many types of medications that can cause water retention. For example: prednisone, non-steroidal anti-inflammatory pills (Voltaren®, Advil®, Naprosyn®, etc), birth control pills, calcium channel blockers (Norvasc®, Cardizem®), Anbrel®, and Remicade® etc.

Polycystic Ovary Syndrome

Polycystic ovaries are found via ultrasound in 21% of premenopausal women. Polycystic ovaries occur due to incomplete follicular development or failure to ovulate. Polycystic ovary syndrome (PCOS) is defined by the occurrence of two of three of the following conditions: high testosterone, anovulatory cycle and ultrasound evidence of polycystic ovary. However, not all of them will develop into PCOS.

PCOS is a common *inherited* disorder (forty percent genetic predisposition) affecting about six percent of women. During the reproductive years, it commonly causes infertility (leading cause of infertility), severe obesity, excessive hair growth, acne, elevated cholesterol and triglycerides, hypertension, and cystic enlargement of the ovaries. . By age fifty, sixty percent of women with PCOS develop Type 2 diabetes since the PCOS gene is in close proximity to the insulin gene on chromosome 19. The diabetes, high cholesterol, obesity, hypertension, and reduced ability to dissolve blood clots secondary to high level of plasminogen activator inhibitor leads to a ten-fold increase in risk of heart attack and stroke. However, only sixty to seventy percent of PCOS patients are obese.

Woman with PCOS have an even higher degree of insulin resistance than those with diabetes. This means that the pancreas must secretes five to ten times more insulin to keep the blood glucose in the normal range. This leads to obesity, water retention, high blood pressure and abnormality in blood lipids. One of the signs of PCOS with insulin resistance is the presence of a thickened skin folds at the back of the neck and is usually darker in color; a condition called *Acanthosis nigricans*. Acanthosis nigricans was first described in PCOS patients in 1976. In severe cases, you may detect multiple skin tags in the neck area. PCOS is also characterized by the over production of male hormones, which come from the enlarged ovaries and adrenal glands. Symptoms of increased male hormones include extra body hair, acne, hypertension, obesity and high cholesterol. The body fat distribution tends to favor the waist area that leads to an "apple-shaped" body. Obese females without PCOS usually have fat at the hip area (pear-shaped). A pear-shaped female may have excess estrogen when compared to their progesterone level. Excessive estrogen promotes fat deposition and cellulite around the hips, thighs and buttocks.

*Note: One may use some natural progesterone products (Wild Yam) and Chromium Picolinate to promote weight loss from the buttocks and thighs.

During the reproductive years, PCOS interferes with the normal release of the pituitary hormones, Luteinizing hormone (LH) and Follicle-stimulating hormone (FSH) which control the ability of the ovary to provide eggs and to produce female hormones. An increase in testosterone from fat increases Gonadotroprin-releasing Hormone (GnRH) secretion that leads to an increase in LH and decrease in FSH. *The LH/FSH ratio is usually >2.* An ovary that is over-stimulated by LH will not mature and therefore the patient cannot ovulate or become pregnant. Eighty percent of females with anovulation have PCOS, and women with PCOS are habitually infertile. A premature egg will diminish estrogen secretion, and increase testosterone secretion. The doctor should check the DHEAs and testosterone level. Testosterone mainly comes from ovary and DHEAs comes from the adrenal gland.

*Note: Brother of PCOS female also has increased testosterone production. However, their DHEAs will be normal. Blocking the androgen receptor with Aldectone® or flutamide improves on insulin sensitivity and decreases the symptoms of PCOS. Small amount of testosterone increase, as in PCOS female, causes fat gain. Large amount of testosterone increase, as in normal male, produces lean muscle mass gain.

Recent research has shown that applying a diabetes management technique to PCOS patient, e.g. taking metformin, Actose® or Avandia® can reduce insulin resistance and hyperinsulinemia (leading to weight reduction), reverse testosterone and LH abnormalities, infertility, and improve the glucose, insulin and lipid profiles.

The classic therapy for symptoms of hyperandrogenism (such as hirsutism and acne) was to suppress ovarian testosterone production with birth control pills. However, the birth control pill can cause weight gain itself. Low dose birth control pills (Allese®, Diane 35®) are better choices. Patients can also augment the estrogenic effect of the birth control pills with the herbs Red Clover and Dong Quai. Spironolactone (Aldectone®) increases the insulin sensitivity by blocking the testosterone effect and diminishes the symptoms of hirsutism.

Case #5. Ms. AM is a 32 year old Italian woman with PCOS, hypertension, gastric reflux, snoring and irregular periods. She weighs 362 pounds and is 5 foot 6 inches tall. Within one year, she *lost 160 pounds*, 16 inches from her waist and 2 inches from her neck. Her blood pressure went down to 95/75. She has regular periods, no more snoring and no reflux symptoms. She did not have to take any medication.

We have many patients who were infertile due to PCOS but later got pregnant after successfully losing their excess weight. It is still safe to continue with this diet during pregnancy while under medical supervision. Obese patients with PCOS are at a higher risk of developing gestational diabetes than normal weight patients.

For normal pregnant patients, the total amount of weight gain should not exceed 28 pounds. Weight increase should be kept to below 6 pounds during the first trimester (3 months), and 11 pounds during the second and third trimesters. Do not increase the calorie intake by more than 100 kcal/day during the first trimester and 200 kcal/day during the subsequent trimesters.

For obese patients, their total weight gain should be less than that of normal weight patients. If she is 120% above her ideal body weight, her total weight gain should not exceed 25 pounds. For 150% above ideal body weight, the total weight gain should be less than 17 pounds[45].

Some people worry that ketones produced during the fat burning process might be harmful to the fetus. It was found that during a normal pregnancy, there is an increase in the rate of lipolysis and ketogenesis during fasting. Ketones can cross across the placenta freely to provide nutrients for the fetus[46]. There is no evidence that physiological ketosis can affect the expecting mother or fetus. In fact, many pregnant women experience morning sickness, which may lead to vomiting and induce ketosis without any harmful effects. Even so, it is common practice to avoid ketosis during pregnancy or breast feeding. May be you can say that we are fear of the "unknown". Hence it is safe to continue with this diet during pregnancy. Since pregnant women will be put on the Phase 2 diet during the pregnancy period, the urine ketone test is negative most of the time. Therefore, it is safe to continue with this diet during pregnancy.

Fatty Liver and Gallstones

The liver is an organ that stores fat readily. As more fat accumulates in the liver, it becomes fatty, a condition known as fatty liver. This disease can be progressive and may lead to elevated liver function test, liver cirrhosis, or liver failure. The definitive diagnosis is through liver biopsy that is seldom done due to the invasiveness of the procedure. Most of the time, routine abdominal ultrasound and liver function tests such as Alanine aminotransferase (ALT) and Aspartame aminotransferase (AST) can detect fatty liver disease. It is more common in an older obese patient who is also suffering from Type 2 diabetes. Individuals with the highest elevations of ALT and AST had significantly greater risk of developing diabetes[47]. CRP and triglycerides levels may also be elevated.

An abnormal liver function test can return to normal once the patient loses weight. People worry that this diet may be bad for the liver. What they do not know is that fatty liver is bad for the liver. Fatty liver is increasingly being diagnosed in those who are overweight, diabetic, or suffering from metabolic syndrome. Study results suggest that insulin sensitizers may be associated with improvements in non-alcoholic steatohepatitis and a reduction in liver disease. More information is forthcoming in the near future[48].

Overweight and obesity are also recognized risk factors for the progression of other chronic liver diseases, such as hepatitis B and C.

Due to the increase in blood cholesterol in obese patients, cholesterol stones are the most common type of "stone" in this group of patients. We once believed that gallstone disease was related to the five "F's": fat, female, fertile, forty, and fair skin. We are now seeing it more common in the obese males and obese teenagers.

***Please note that for any person who changes his/her diet radically the chance of gallstone formation is increased. This applies to both starting and stopping a diet program.

Osteoarthritis

The most common areas of musculoskeletal pain in the obese population are the knees, hips and lower back in descending order. Osteoarthritis is the usual pathology. The knee and hip joints are called the weight bearing joints and can only handle a certain amount of weight. As the patient gains weight, there is extra stress put on these points and the grinding force on the joints causes damage, first to the hyaline cartilage, and eventually to the bones themselves.

The natural history of osteoarthritis of the knee joint starts with stiffness and pain to the knee during weight bearing activities, such as walking. Once the cartilage wears out, often unevenly between the two halves of the knee joint, there will be an angle deformity at the knee joint leading to the formation of bowlegs or knock-knees, depending on which side of the knee joint wears out first. The ligaments that hold the knee together get stretched and produce pain. Inflammation of the joint causes redness, heat, pain, swelling (increase synovial fluid) and thickening of the synovial membrane. It makes knee bending more difficult. Because of pain and stiffness, the patient usually tends not to move the knee as much, leading to muscle wasting. If nothing is done to stop the progression of the disease, the patient will have constant pain, even during sleep, and will be required to have a total knee replacement surgery (arthroplasty). The same situation is true with osteoarthritis of the hip. The destructive process of the hip joint is due to excessive stress on the joint surface. The pain is usually located at the groin area or to the front part of the thigh. If the osteoarthritis is due to obesity, it makes sense to minimize the progression of the disease through weight loss. Even if it is too late to prevent total knee arthroplasty, it is imperative to lose weight before surgery and to prevent osteoarthritis on the opposite side. It is not unusual to find a patient suffering from both knee and hip arthritis and have both knees and hips replaced. The synthetic components of the arthroplasty are supposed to last for twenty years. However, the obese patient constantly puts more stress on the artificial joints and promotes quicker destruction of the artificial joints.

Osteoarthritis of the back is very common in the adult population. However, studies have failed to link back pain with obesity. That is not to say that obesity does not cause back pain. However, if the patient has low back pain already for whatever reason, the obese patient will have more symptoms. The symptoms will subside with weight reduction.

Sleep Apnea and Respiratory Problems

Sleep apnea means that there is a stoppage of breathing for more than ten seconds at a time and this occurs at least five times per hour. There are two kinds of sleep apnea - obstructive and non-obstructive (central) sleep apnea. The only sure way to diagnose central sleep apnea is to demonstrate significant desaturation in a sleep study. The major risk factor for obstructive sleep apnea is obesity. Seventy to eighty percent of all new cases are significantly overweight. In people with a body mass index of 30 or more, 20-30% turns out to have obstructive sleep apnea and 50% of those with a BMI over 40 have the condition. Twenty-four percent of adult men and nine percent of adult women are estimated to have some degree of obstructive sleep apnea (collapse of the upper airway).

One or more of the following symptoms may be noted with sleep apnea:

- Sleepiness and fatigue. Due to repetitive arousal, sleep fragmentation, and lack of oxygen to the brain during sleep apnea, there may be a decline in performance on the job, in school, or while driving. This increases the patient's risk of a motor vehicle accident. Hence, a physician must notify the Ministry of Transportation of the patient's severe sleep apnea and suspend the driving license until the condition is properly treated.

- Memory loss

- Depression, irritability and mood swing

- Dry or sore throat on awakening

- Restless sleep

- Night sweat

- Snoring

- Hypertension

- Congestive heart failure

Risk factors of sleep apnea:

- Obesity, particularly upper body obesity, is a risk factor for sleep apnea and has been shown to relate to its severity. The major pathophysiologic consequences of severe sleep apnea include arterial hypoxemia (lack of oxygen), recurrent arousal from sleep, increased sympathetic tone, pulmonary and systemic hypertension, and cardiac arrhythmia. Most people with sleep apnea have a BMI of more than 30.

- Short and thick neck. Large neck girth in both men and women who snore is highly predictive of sleep apnea. In general, men whose neck circumference is 17 inches or greater and women whose neck circumference is 16 inches or greater are at higher risk for sleep apnea[49].

- Deviated nasal septum

- Broad face; small jaw

- Long soft palate; thick tongue

- Enlarged tonsils and adenoids (especially children)

Life style changes might improve the symptoms of sleep apnea:

- Change sleeping habits - sleeping on one's side instead of on one's back

- Weight loss

- Avoid alcohol, smoking, sleeping pills and tranquilizers. These agents can cause the throat tissue to sag and restrict breathing.

If these fail, one can try sleeping with a Continuous Positive Airflow Pressure (CPAP) machine, mandibular advancement devices, or surgery (e.g. uvulopalatopharyngoplasty, nasal surgery, tonsillectomy etc.).

Obese patients often complain that they have shortness of breath. It takes much effort for them to take a deep breath, and therefore they usually take shallow breaths. Because of abdominal obesity, there is an increase in the intra-abdominal pressure and the diaphragm has difficulty in moving downward during inspiration. Obesity can also cause chest wall stiffness and make it difficult to deeply inhale or fully exhale. This leads to low blood oxygen and high blood carbon dioxide levels. *Pickwickian Syndrome* is due to end-stage respiratory failure secondary to obesity where the patient breathes very shallow and feels sleepy all the time. This can progress into heart failure.

There may be optimal sleeping hours at which body weight regulation is facilitated. Indeed, short sleep duration predicts an increased risk of being overweight or obese in adults. Lack of sleep is related to a reduction of circulating leptin level relative to what is predicted by the fat mass. Sleep deprivation result in changes in levels of several hormones including leptin, ghrelin, insulin, cortisol, and growth hormone. These hormonal changes may contribute to energy imbalance and then lead to overweight or obesity[50].

Hyperuricemia

Elevated serum uric acid level is common in an obese individual. It is also loosely related to people suffering from metabolic syndrome (Chapter 5). Uric acid is a waste product of protein metabolism. It is also found in large quantities in some foods (Table 15). An elevated uric acid level in blood does not necessary cause disease. An asymptomatic high uric acid level (hyperuricemia) per se does not require therapy. However when uric acid crystallizes in urine, uric acid stone is formed. Gout is a type of inflammatory arthritis when uric acid crystallizes in the joints, especially the big toe, ankle or knee. It is more common in males than females.

Dehydration, acidic urine, or a sudden uric acid load can trigger the formation of uric acid stone or gout. This means that what you eat and drink directly affects your chance of gout attack.

If you have a history of uric acid stone or gout, you need to drink enough water to pass pale urine consistently. Keep the urine pH to about 6.5 to 7 with medication (potassium citrate 30-60 mmol/day in divided doses) if necessary. Do not raise the pH above 7 because it can cause calcium stones to form. Avoid foods that are high in uric acid precursor (purine). Avoid excessive alcohol, especially beer. If the serum uric acid remains high (over 600 mmol/L in female or over 750 mmol/L in male) you may need to take 100 to 300 mg of allopurinol per day.

Table 15. Foods high in purine (uric acid).	
Shellfish	Lobster, Mussel
Organ meat	Liver, Kidney, Brains, Sweetbreads
Red meat	Any Red Meat
Vegetables	Peas, Beans
Fish	Anchovies, Mackerel, Sardines, Herring

High uric acid levels can also be due to taking diuretic medications (water pills). Commonly used diuretics are Lasix® (furosemide), Triazide® (triamterene/hydrochlorothiazide), hydrochlorothiazide, Moduret® (hydrochlorothiazide/amiloride hydrochloride), and Lozide® (indapamide hemihydrate). Aldactone® (spironolactone) is the exception; it does not elevate serum uric acid level. Another type of medication typically used in transplant patients called Cyclosporine has been associated with severe hyperuricemia and gout. Hyperuricemia is also common in patients with chronic renal (kidney) failure and lymphoproliferative disorders. High uric acid in patients less than 30 years old can be secondary to genetic factors.

Fructose intake has been implicated in causing hyperuricemia.

Gout usually occurs at the big toe. It can also occur at the instep, ankle, heel, knee, wrist, finger, and elbow. Gout can occur within hours, usually starting at middle of the night. Triggering factors of acute gout attack can be from direct trauma (e.g. minor sprain toe or ankle), long walks, excessive alcohol consumption, surgery, over eating, starvation, or taking diuretics.

Fibromyalgia and Chronic Fatigue Syndrome

It has not been until recently that fibromyalgia and chronic fatigue syndromes are recognized as a medical illness. Unlike diabetes or rheumatoid arthritis, there are no tests to diagnose these diseases. Hence, these patients are usually misdiagnosed with depression or considered lazy. This is a list of symptoms common in patients suffering from chronic fatigue syndrome.

- Tender spots and morning stiffness on muscles all over the body

- Fatigue, depression, anxiety, insomnia, impaired concentration

- Irritable bowel

- Frequent urination, dysuria (burning urination)

- Skin rash (hives, eczema)

- Headache, vertigo

- Hypoglycemia (low blood sugar)

Two to seven percent of the population has fibromyalgia. This is predominantly a female disease (85%), most common in the 30 to 55 age group when the symptoms first begin. What causes fibromyalgia? Some say it is due to excessive accumulation of phosphate in the cells. Some say it is due to a viral infection. Some say it is inherited. Alternatively, is it due to physical and/or mental trauma? Since the disease does not respond to prednisone treatment, fibromyalgia may not be an inflammatory disease. With chronic pain, sleep dysfunction and fatigue, patients have a very low amount of physical activity. Hypoglycemic syndrome is associated with 40% of patients suffering from fibromyalgia. With the hypoglycemia, the patient will be eating high carbohydrate meals in order to relieve the symptoms, not knowing that it can cause more hypoglycemic episodes two hours later. They become obese due to the over consumption of carbohydrates. Treatment of this disease is usually symptomatic. Doctors treat psychological problems with antidepressants (which may cause weight gain), the muscle pain stiffness with pain medications and the bowel problems with motility modifying drugs. Most of these treatment options are not very effective. Some suggest using guaifenesin (an expectorant for colds medication) to block the re-absorption of phosphate in the kidneys. Very often, a patient with fibromyalgia also suffers from hypoglycemia. The symptoms are very similar. Patients should be put on a low carbohydrate diet that should solve the problem of hypoglycemia and obesity. The symptoms of fibromyalgia may also get better.

Although patients who are obese and suffering from fibromyalgia have less activity than the normal population, it is important to push this type of patient to do cardiovascular exercises. Studies have shown that aerobic exercises improve pain symptoms and diminish depression. The same benefit was not demonstrated with weight training.

References:

1. Knowler WC, Barrett-Connor E, Fowler SE, et al. Reduction in the incidence of Type 2 diabetes with lifestyle intervention or metformin. N Engl J Med 2002;346:393-403.

2. Tuomilehto J, Lindstrom J, Eriksson JG, et al. Prevention of Type 2 diabetic mellitus by changes in lifestyle among subjects with impaired glucose tolerance. N Engl J Med 2001;344:1345-1350.

3. Wing RR, Marcus MD, Epstein LH, et al. Type 2 diabetic subjects lose less weight than their overweight non-diabetic spouses. Diabetes Care 1987;10:563-566.

4. Boden G, Jadall F, White J, et al. Effects of fat on insulin-stimulated carbohydrate metabolism in normal men. J Clin Invest 1991;88(3):960-6.

5. Boden G, Chen X, Ruiz J, et al. Mechanisms of fatty acid-induced inhibition of glucose uptake. J Clin Invest 1994;93:2438-46.

6. Fitchett D. Dysglycemia in the Patient with Coronary Artery Disease: An Often Unrecognized Modifiable Risk Factor. Metabolic Syndrome Rounds December 2005.

7. Coughlin CC, Finck BN, Eagon C, et al. Obesity 2007;15:640-45.

8. Arita Y, et al. Paradoxical decrease of an adipose-specific protein, adiponectin, in obesity. Biochem Biophys Res Common 1999;257:79.

9. Lindsay RS, et al. Adiponectin and development of type 2 diabetes in the Pima Indian population. Lancet 2002;360:57-58.

10. Phillips SA, et al. Modulation of circulating and adipose tissue adiponectin levels by antidiabetic therapy. Diabetes 2003;52:667-674.

11. Simpson SH, Majumdar SR, Tsuyuki RT, et al. Dose-response relation between sulfonylurea drugs and mortality in Type 2 diabetes mellitus: a population-based cohort study. CMAJ 2006;174(2):169-74.

12. McCormack J, Johns K, Tildesley H. Metformin's countraindications should be contraindicated. CMAJ 2005;173:502-504.

13. Poon P, Poon D, Wong M, Endogenous Insulin Production in Obese NIDDM Patients taking Insulin. Obesity 2008;16supp:S251.

14. Khan MA, Gannon MC, Nuttall FQ. Glucose appearance rate following protein ingestion in normal subjects. J Am Coll Nutr 1992;11:701-706.

15. Nuttall FQ, Gannon MC. Plasma glucose and insulin response to macronutrients in nondiabetics and TYPE 2 DIABETIC subjects. Diabetes Care 1991;14:824-38.

16. Leiter LA, Yale JF, Chiasson JL, et al. Assessment of the impact of fear of hypoglycemic episodes on glycemic and hypoglycemia management. Can J Diabetes 2005;29:186-192.

17. UK Prospective Diabetes Study Group. UK Prospective Diabetes Study 16. Overview of 6 years' therapy of Type II diabetes: a progressive disease. Diabetes 1995;44:1249-58.

18. Robyn L. Houlden, Treating the Spikes: Is Targeting Postprandial Hyperglycemia Important in Type 2 Diabetes? Canadian Diabetes 2007;20:3-5.

19. Dahlof B, Sever PSk Poulter NR, et al. Prevention of cardiovascular events with an antihypertensive regimen of amlodipine adding perindopril as required versus atenolol adding bendroflumethiazide as required in the ASCOT-BPLA: A multicentre randomised controlled trial. Lancet 2005;366:895-906.

20. Leibowitz G, Yuli M, Donath MY, et al. Beta-cell glucotoxicity in the Psammomys obesus model of Type 2 diabetes. Diabetes 2001;50:S113-7.

21. Turner RC, Cull CA, Frighi V, et al. Glycemic control with diet, sulfonylurea, metformin, or insulin in patients with Type 2 diabetes mellitus: progressive requirement for multiple therapies. JAMA 1999;281:2005-15.

22. McGarry JD. Banting Lecture 2001: Dysregulation of fatty acid metabolism in the etiology of Type 2 diabetes. Diabetes 2002;51:7-18.

23. Stratton IM, Adler AI, Neil HAW, et al. Association of glycemia with macrovascular and microvascular complications of Type 2 diabetes: prospective observational study. JAMA 2000;321:405-12.

24. Leahy JL, Meir GC. Evolution of abnormal insulin secretary responses during 48-h in vivo hyperglycemia. Diabetes 1988;37 (2):217-22.

25. Leahy JL, Bonner-Weir S, Weir GC. Minimal chronic hyperglycemia is a critical determinant of impaired insulin secretion after an incomplete pancreatectomy. J Clin Invest 1988;81(5);1407-14.

26. Kelley DE, Mandarino LJ. Fuel selection in human skeletal muscle in insulin resistance: a reexamination. Diabetes 2000;49(5):677-83.

27. Villareal D, Banks M, Patterson B, et al. Weight Loss Therapy Improves Pancreatic Endocrine Function in Obese Older Adults. Obesity 2008;16:1349-54.

28. Wassmann S, Stumpf M, Strehlow K, et al. Interleukin-6 induces oxidative stress and endothelial dysfunction by over-expression of the angiotensin II Type 1 receptor. Circ Res 2004;94:534-41.

29. Kern PA, Saghizadeh M, et al. The expression of tumor necrosis factor in human adipose tissue. Regulation by obesity, weight loss and relationship to lipoprotein lipase. J Clin Invest 1995;95:2111-9.

30. Yesilbursa D, Serdar A, et al. The effect of orlistat-induced weight loss on interleukin-6 and C-reactive protein levels in obese objects. Acta Cardiol 2005;60:265-9.

31. Arita Y, et al. Paradoxical decrease of an adipose-specific protein, adiponectin, in obesity. Biochem Biophys Res Commun 1999;257:79-83.

32. Lindsay RS, et al. Adiponectin and development of Type 2 diabetes in Pima Indian population. Lancet 2002;360:57-8.

33. Phillips SA, et al. Modulation of circulating and adipose tissue adiponectin levels by anti-diabetic therapy. Diabetes 2003;52:667-74.

34. Gannon MC et al. An increase in dietary protein improves the blood glucose response in persons with Type 2 diabetes. Am J Clin Nutr 2003;78:734-741.

35. Eckel RH. A new look at dietary protein in diabetes. Am J Clin Nutr 2003;78:671-672.

36. Landsberg L, Young JB. Insulin-mediated glucose metabolism in the relationship between dietary intake and sympathetic nervous system activity. International J Obesity 1985;9:63-68.

37. Bigazzi R, Bianchi S, Baldari G, Campese VM. Clustering of cardiovascular risk factors in salt-sensitive patients with essential hypertension: role of insulin. Am J Hypertension 1996;9:24-32.

38. Randeree HA, Omar MA, Motala AA, Seedat MA. Effect of insulin therapy on blood pressure in TYPE 2 DIABETIC patients with secondary failure. Diabetes Care 1992;15:1258-1263.

39. Tedde R, Sechi LA, Marigliano A, et al. Antihypertensive effect of insulin reduction in diabetic-hypertensive patients. Am J Hypertension 1989;2:163-170.

40. Shirya R, Jacques G. Effect of obesity on high-density lipoprotein metabolism. Obesity 2007; 15:2875-88.

41. Genest et al. Recommendations for the management of dyslipidemia and the prevention of cardiovascular disease: 2003 update. CMAJ 2003;169(9):921-924.

42. Stanhope KL, Schwarz JM, Keim NL, et al. Consuming fructose-sweetened, not glucose-sweetened, beverages increases visceral adiposity and lipids and decreases insulin sensitivity in overweight/obese humans. J. Clin. Invest 2009:10:1172.

43. Wassmann S, Stumpf M, Strehlow K, et al. Interleukin-6 induces oxidative stress and endothelial dysfunction by overexpression of the angiotensin II type 1 receptor. Circ Res 2004;94:534-541.

44. Cheryan M. Phytic acid interactions in food systems. Crit Rev Food Sci Nutr 1980;13:297-335.

45. Meltzer SJ. Management of diabetes in pregnancy: Challenges and Trends. Can J Diabetes 2005;29(3):246-56.

46. Freinkel N. Benting Lecture 1980. Of pregnancy and progeny. Diabetes 1980;29:1023-35.

47. Hanley AJ, Williams K, Festa A, et al. Elevations in markers of liver injury and risk of type 2 diabetes: the insulin resistance atherosclerosis study. Diabetes 2005;53:2623-32.

48. Tilg H, Kaser A. Treatment strategies in nonalcoholic fatty liver disease. Nat Clin Pract Gastroenterol Hepatol 2005;2:148-55.

49. Davies RJ et al. The relationship between neck circumference, radiographic pharyngeal anatomy, and the obstructive sleep apnea syndrome. Eur Respir J 1990;3:509-514.

50. Xiaoli Chen, May Beydoun and Youfa Wang. Is sleep duration associated with childhood obesity? A systematic review and meta-analysis. Obesity 2008; 16:265-74.

*"Thou should not weight more than
the refrigerator."*

4: CHILDHOOD OBESITY

Whatever the cause, there is a steady rise in childhood obesity in North America. Ten to fifteen percent of the children in U.S. are overweight. Since the gene pool did not change much in the last century, the change in food consumption behavior (increase in consumption of fast foods, soda and juice) by our children is likely the cause of the increased prevalence of obesity. Due to computer games, television and television games children expend much less energy.

One of the most commonly used methods to assess if a child is obese is to measure the child's BMI. Using the gender specific growth charts invented by the United States Centers for Disease Control and Prevention, compare the child's BMI is compared with that of his/her peers. If the BMI falls between the 85th to 95th percentiles, the child is overweight. If the BMI is over the 95th percentile, the child is obese.

There are risks associated with childhood obesity:

1. Social and psychological effects. Overweight children may develop low self-esteem, depression, anxiety, difficulty with relationships, and face discrimination in social situations

2. Hypertension

3. High cholesterol and triglycerides. Rapid weight gain in the early teen years can damage the heart by early adulthood

4. Type 2 diabetes and hyperinsulinemia. This is different from Type 1 diabetes in that Type 2 diabetes has elevated fasting insulin and C-peptide levels

5. Fatty liver. There is elevation of the serum alanine aminotransferase (ALT) level, which will come down with modest weight loss

6. Headaches. Doctor may need to rule out pseudotumor cerebri. This occurs more frequently in young females. It is caused by an increase in cranial pressure leading to intracranial hypertension. Although the CT scan will be normal, the patient develops headaches and blurred vision

7. Slipped femoral capital epiphysis and Blount disease (Tibia Vara). Obese children put excessive weight on the femoral head (hipbone) and cause the growth plate to slip. They will have pain in the hip area. Children with Blount disease will present with bowed legs and complain of pain to the inside of the tibia just below the knee

8. Snoring and sleep apnea. Pay extra attention if tonsillectomy fails to correct the problem. The child needs weight reduction

9. Acne

10. Irregular period such as missing period and PCOS

It is safe for children and adolescents to go on this diet. The child's exercise program may have to be modified, as extreme weight training is contra-indicated in a growing child.

Sometimes the parents need counseling because they are the ones who feed their children. What they think is healthy for their children may actually cause the children to become obese.

Products advertised as *"made with real fruits"* or fruit drinks labeled with *"contains 30% real fruit juice"* actually have a very high sugar content. Advertisers make use of the general misconception that "fruit and juice are good for you." Fruit and juice are healthy foods if you do not need to lose weight. When your grandparents and your parents keep on telling you the same message repeatedly that juice is good for you, you accept that as the truth. You then pass on the message to your own children. Even the World Health Organization (WHO) has associated fruit juice with obesity in its report, entitled "Diet, Nutrition, and the Prevention of Chronic Diseases." WHO also wants the government to take steps to limit children's exposure to junk-food advertising and says that added sugar should comprise no more than 10% of a healthy diet. By calculation, recommendations given by the Canada Food Guide for Healthy Eating can add up to 12% sugar per day. The report continues to state that each additional can or glass of sugar-sweetened drink consumed every day increases the risk of becoming obese by 60%. Most of the evidence relates to soda drinks but many fruit drinks and sport drinks are equally energy-dense and may promote weight gain if consumed in large quantities. The name of the sugar that is present in fruit juice is sucrose. Sucrose is a disaccharide consisting of one glucose molecule and one fructose molecule in equal portions. The increased in the consumption of fructose has been linked to the increased in the prevalence of obesity in the past two to three decades[1-2].

In a study, fructose-sweetened beverages were shown to increase obesity in animal study[3]. Fructose has a lower glycemic index than glucose but it does not trigger the secretion of insulin or leptin. Leptin is secreted from the stomach in response to food ingestion to trigger satiety. If fructose does not induce the leptin secretion after ingestion, it may contribute to increased caloric intake. A child who drinks juice may not know when to stop drinking because the type of sugar in juice does not trigger the satiety response in the central nervous system.

Most people agree that potato chips are junk food. However many people feed their children mashed potatoes with gravy. Is mashed potato with gravy really better than potato chips?

Children learn by observing their parents. The environment that parents create, by way of their own dietary and physical activity behavior may have a lasting negative effect on their children's weight trajectories and their emerging obesity risk behaviors, such as their dietary patterns[4]. Whatever you eat, they will consider as the norm. You have to lead by example. You cannot tell your children not to smoke if you continue to smoke.

Patients always tell me that obesity runs in their family and it must be genetic. Yes, it is possible, but not probable. Since the whole family eats the same food, if the type of diet makes the father fat, the same type of food will make the son fat also.

If you are suffering from diabetes, hypertension, or coronary heart disease, your children are prone to the same diseases if they are obese. You can minimize their risk by controlling their weight. A study done by Dr. Gerald Schulman of the Yale University School of Medicine demonstrated that children of diabetic parents are more prone to develop diabetes even when they are not as fat as the children of non-diabetic parents are. It may be due to decreased activity of muscle mitochondria that leads to a decrease in energy output and increase in the fat buildup in the muscle cells. Since there is a strong relationship between fat content in the muscle and insulin resistance, and insulin resistance is the best predicator of whether someone will eventually develop Type 2 diabetes, these children are more prone to becoming diabetic if they gain fat weight.

The school cafeteria needs to be more health-conscious. I am happy that some of Toronto's grade schools are beginning to serve healthier meals. Instead of poutine, one school is serving Caesar salad and chicken burgers. Not the best choice, but it is a start.

If you go to your local hospital and visit the cafeteria, how many will be selling muffins, pizza and French fries! My local hospital has vending machines selling chips, pop, candies and trans fat laden cookies. Is the hospital looking for more business? This hospital is built right across from a high school. Students come to the hospital cafeteria to buy their lunches. There is a popular combo that they like. It consists of a bottle of pop, one slice of pizza and a bag of chips.

Obese school children in New South Wales, Australia who are obese ate more veggies and fruits per day than non-obese children did. Hence just by telling our children to eat more fruit and vegetables is not the solution[5]. According to USDA surveys, in 1965 white potato accounted for one third of all vegetable intake by children, whereas by 1996, potato accounted for half of all vegetable consumption[6]. A 2-year school-based weight prevention project in Louisiana employs a diet that is lower in calories by limiting fat and protein and increasing physical activity; however, this did not result in any change in weight[7]. When these school children were put on a low fat and protein diet, in order to achieve the total daily calorie intake requirement, they were eating more carbohydrates.

Parents have to increase their children's level of activity through participation in organized sports. House league sports are usually non-competitive and highly enjoyable. The message here is to participate, winning is secondary. Encourage them to join sports clubs at school. Do not feed the overweight children high carbohydrate foods or drinks after the sporting events. This will defeat the purpose of exercise.

Study after study has shown that in order for children to lose weight, a combination of diet and moderate exercise is needed. Experts agree that this type of diet can get children to lose weight quickly and that it can be done safely with the help of a professional. However, without increased activity, the long-term success rate is low. Hence, before accepting any children into any diet program make sure that they are willing to do the extra activity. Otherwise, the program is doomed to fail. Calcium and potassium supplementation may be needed just as with adults, especially if they sweat a lot during exercise.

Positive reinforcement will be helpful. Any weight reduction should be viewed as an accomplishment. The whole family may need to change their eating habits and activity pattern in order to help the child. Parents and physicians should encourage and not criticize even if the child fails to lose weight. Do not use food as a "reward" to treat the child!

Encourage the child to eat small frequent meals. The prevalence of obesity is decreased by the number of daily meals[8].

Pay attention to those children who are not really overweight but insist on dieting. These are the children who are prone to developing an eating disorder.

References:

1. Elliott SS, et al. Fructose, weight gain, and the insulin resistance syndrome. Am J Clin Nutr 2002;76:911-922.

2. Bray GA, et al. Consumption of high-fructose corn syrup in beverages may play a role in the epidemic of obesity. Am J Clin Nutr 2004;79:537-543.

3. Jurgens H, et al. Consuming fructose-sweetened beverages increases body adiposity in mice. Obesity Research 2005;13:1146-1156.

4. Davison KK, Francis La, Birch LL. Reexamining Obesigenic Families: Parents' Obesity-related Behaviors Predict Girls' Change in BMI. Obesity Research 2005;11:1980-90.

5. Elizabeth Denney-Wilson, et al. Healthy Food Habits and Fitness: A solution to the metabolic risk factors associated with overweight in adolescents? Obesity Research Sept 2005 vol 13. Program abstract supplement A30.

6. Cavadini C, Siega-Riz AM, Popkin BM. West J Med 2000;173:378-83.

7. Williamson D, Copeland A, Anton S, et al. Wise Mind Project: A school-based environmental approach fro preventing weight gain in children. Obesity 2007;15:906-17.

8. Toschke AM, Kuchenhoff H, Koletzko B. Meal frequency and Childhood Obesity. Obesity Research 2005;11:1932-38.

"I would give up chocolate but I'm no QUITTER."

5 : Metabolic Syndrome

As a teenager, Mr. P was an average height and weight. He participated in many extra-curricular activities such as soccer, basketball, and martial arts. Even though he ate quite a bit, he did not get fat.

While at university, Mr. P worked in the cafeteria and the food was free. He started to overeat. As the workload of his studies got busier, there was less time for exercise. He began to gain weight.

During graduate school, Mr. P stopped overeating and he began to exercise. He was engaged to be married and the wedding was to happen right after he finished graduate school. He wanted to look his best for the wedding. That was over thirty years ago. Once he got married, his weight went up steadily. He did not particularly over eat but he would eat everything served to him. He did play badminton, but not consistently enough.

His weight was almost 176 pounds (80kg), his waist circumference was 103 cm, body mass index was 30 (class 1 obesity), and percentage of body fat was 29%. He had headaches and lower back pain. His wife told him that he snored loudly. He had hypertension and although he took three different antihypertensive medications, his blood pressure was still high (130/95).

Mr. P's fasting blood glucose was 6.7 mmol/L (normal range is 3.6-6.0 mmol/L for Canadians) which told him that he was at risk for future development of Type 2 diabetes.

Mr. P's cholesterol was high at 6.48 mmol/L and triglycerides was on the high side (2.88 mmol/L). His LDL cholesterol (bad cholesterol) was 4.09 mmol/L. A patient with a LDL cholesterol level of greater than 3.4 mmol/L carries a higher risk of coronary heart disease. His HDL cholesterol (good cholesterol) was 1.08 mmol/L, which was on the low side of normal. One wants the HDL to be as high as possible. A more sensitive index to predict coronary heart disease is called the Cholesterol to HDL ratio. Normal is anything less than 5 and his was 6.

Fatty liver is a term that a doctor gives to a patient with an enlarged liver and abnormal serum liver enzyme tests. It is an index of obesity. Two out of three liver function tests on his blood work showed mild elevation, which indicated that his liver was fatty. By itself, fatty liver is usually harmless. However, it gives an indirect signal that one is obese. Occasionally, it can lead to cirrhosis.

There are many definition of *Metabolic Syndrome*. The most commonly used definition in Canada is the one given by the National Cholesterol Education Program Adult Treatment Panel III. It defines Metabolic Syndrome as a cluster of at least three of the following five signs, abdominal obesity, high blood glucose (impaired fasting glucose, impaired glucose tolerance, insulin resistance, or diabetes), high serum triglycerides, low HDL cholesterol, and high blood pressure (Table 16). When we say that a patient is suffering from Metabolic Syndrome, we mean that there is an imbalance in the patient's anabolic and catabolic pathways. Patients accumulate fat, this leads to hypertension, dyslipidemia and eventually diabetes.

Table 16. Definition of Metabolic Syndrome.	
According to National Cholesterol Education Program Adult Treatment Panel III: Metabolic Syndrome is present when the patient has three of the following five criteria:	
1. Abdominal obesity (waist circumference)	> 102 cm for male > 88 cm for female
2. Fasting blood glucose	> 6.0 mmol/L*
3. Triglycerides	> 1.7mmol/L*
4. HDL cholesterol	< 1.0 mmol/L* for male < 1.3 mmol/L* for female
5. Blood pressure	> 130/85*

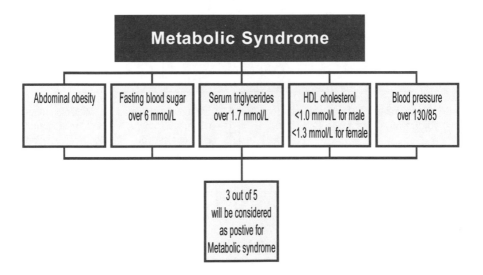

According to the World Health Organization, Metabolic Syndrome is present when the patient has impaired fasting glucose, impaired glucose tolerance or diabetes, plus two of the following four criteria:	
1. Waist-to-hip ratio	> 0.85 for female or > 0.9 for male or BMI > 30
2. Triglycerides	> 1.7 mmol/L* and/or HDL cholesterol < 1.0 mmol/L*
3. Blood pressure	> 140/90*
4. Microalbuminuria	> 20 microgram/min* or albumin/creatinine ratio > 30 mg/g*

* Untreated values

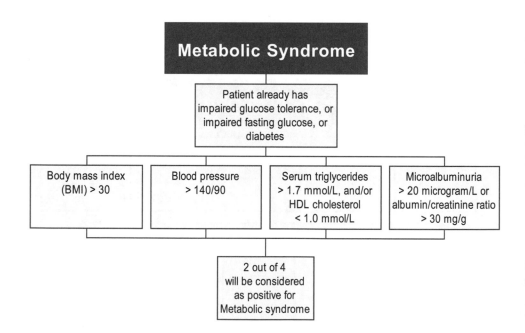

According to the International Diabetes Federation (2006), in order to be suffering from Metabolic Syndrome, the patient has to be obese. That is, if the patient is not obese, the patient cannot have Metabolic Syndrome:

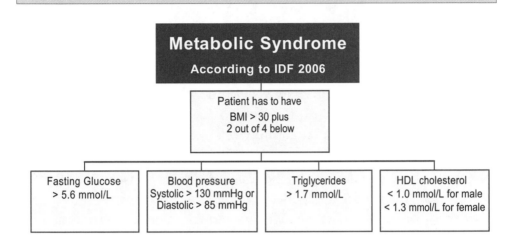

Another definition of Metabolic Syndrome, but not as popular, was provided by the World Health Organization. It stated that the patient has to have an abnormal blood glucose test first, and two out of four other symptoms to considered as suffering from Metabolic Syndrome. I do not like this definition because out of all the symptoms of Metabolic Syndrome, diabetes usually comes last. If the patient has to show an abnormal blood glucose test first, there is a good chance that the patient will already developed dyslipidemia or hypertension. One of the reasons to label a patient with Metabolic Syndrome is to provide early interventions such as diet, exercise or medications so that the patient may not develop the full blown disease.

The latest definition of Metabolic Syndrome, which happens to be my favorite one, is proposed by the International Diabetic Federation in 2006. It states that obesity is the root of all evils. Without obesity, a patient will not develop Metabolic Syndrome. Hence, it is important to screen all obese patients for signs of Metabolic Syndrome.

The International Diabetes Federation also stated that for patients with a BMI of over 30, there is no need to measure the waist circumference. This means that there is only a very small chance that when the patient is obese according to the BMI reading, the patient is not centrally obese. Obese patients cannot be overweight in muscle and not fat.

In October 2005, the American Heart Association and the National Heart, Lung, and Blood Institute published the modified National Cholesterol Education Program's definition of Metabolic Syndrome with the same lowered cutoff-point for fasting glucose and ethnic-specific criteria for weight circumfences[1].

No matter how you define Metabolic Syndrome, a consensus exists that there is a strong linkage between Metabolic Syndrome and family history of insulin resistance. Weight reduction and exercise are the cornerstones of lifestyle modification for the prevention and treatment of Metabolic Syndrome.

According to the WHO, 300 million people in the world are obese and there are potentially 21 million of patients suffering from Metabolic Syndrome. The study of a group of men aged 42 to 60, over a 15-year period found that those with Metabolic Syndrome were 2.9 to 4.2 times more likely to die of a heart attack than those who did not have the condition. Metabolic Syndrome is also associated with subsequent development of arteriosclerosis, fatty liver, elevated uric acid level, Type 2 diabetes, renal disease and blood clots. The Centers for Disease Control and Prevention estimates that one in five adults in North America already has metabolic syndrome and that the numbers will continue to grow because of the North Americans' sedentary lifestyle. It looked like Mr. P was heading in that direction.

The use of Metabolic Syndrome in predicting the patient's diabetic risk is 4-fold more sensitive than it is for predicting coronary heart disease. The risk of developing of coronary heart disease is highest in patients with Metabolic Syndrome and diabetes, less for those who have

Metabolic Syndrome without diabetes and even less for patients with diabetes without Metabolic Syndrome.

We find that it is difficult to measure the waist circumference or the waist-to-hip ratio accurately. It is also difficult to reproduce the results week after week. There are ethnic differences regarding the waist to hip ratios. Orientals tend to have a smaller gluteal muscle as compared to a person of African origin. The waist-to-hip ratio will be artificially high in the oriental population. We prefer to use the BMI or the percentage of body fat as the method of choice in estimating obesity.

It did not matter which definition was used, Mr. P had Metabolic Syndrome. After adding up the points according to Table 14, he scored a total of 12 points, and his 10-year risk was 10%. However, because his father had diabetes and stroke, and his sister also has metabolic syndrome, he should multiply his 10-year risk by two, which increases his risk to 20%. His targets for LDL cholesterol should be less than 2.5 mmol/L and total cholesterol to HDL cholesterol ratio should be less than 4.0. As shown above, Mr. P's blood levels were higher than the target values.

Mr. P also noticed that in one of the pictures he took during a recent holiday, his belly was bulging. He decided that he needed to do something about it. Rather than medications, he opted for lifestyle changes. He picked a day to start his diet. He told himself that *no one could help him if he did not help himself first*. His family was very supportive and his wife prepared his meals according to this diet plan.

During the early years of his career, he was working many hours a day and sometimes 36 hours straight. This put too much stress on his body. He quit one of his jobs that involved being on-call 24 hours a day so that he could have undisturbed sleep.

Mr. P followed this diet plan without deviation. Although he was allowed to have more carbohydrates after the Induction Phase (Phase

1), He tried not to increase his carbohydrate load. At the same time, he started to exercise at the gym. He spent about 3 hours per week doing weight training and jogging on the treadmill.

At the end of eight weeks, he lost 24 pounds (11 kg), which was equal to a 14% drop of his weight. His percentage of body fat came down to 19% (22% is acceptable). His body mass index came down to 26 (27 is acceptable, 25 is normal), which was equal to a drop of 10%. He dropped three inches from his waistline at this point. It looked like he had reached his goal and he started to eat according to the Maintenance Phase (Phase 3). His weight remained the same for 1 month. During this month, he did not have any ketones in the urine.

The development of Metabolic Syndrome is partly genetic (runs in the family), partly environmental (obesity from overeating or eating the wrong diet), or lifestyle (sedentary). Since there is nothing we can do about the genetic factor, weight loss and increased physical activities are the cornerstones of treating Metabolic Syndrome. However, do not hesitate to use medications to control the hypertension, glucose intolerance, or the abnormal lipid profile until the diet and exercise program starts to take effect. The main idea is to prevent coronary heart disease, stroke, blindness, or renal disease, just to mention a few.

Later, Mr. P wished to lose more fat and he went back to the Induction Phase. After three days of a protein and vegetable only diet, he began to detect ketones in the urine again. He did sit-ups and push-ups everyday and he jogged five kilometers twice weekly. On week fourteen, he succeeded in lowering his body mass index to 25 and decreased the percentage of body fat to 18%. He lost another inch from his waistline.

Without any antihypertensive medications, his average blood pressure is now 118/78 (according to the 24-hour ambulatory blood pressure monitoring). His headache has gone away. According to his wife, he does not snore anymore.

His eighteen-month post-diet blood work shows great improvement (Table 17). The results showed that he no longer suffers from impair fasting glucose (even though he will always be at risk). His risk for having coronary heart disease has been lowered significantly as shown by the normal total cholesterol to HDL cholesterol ratio. His liver function tests (AST, GGT) have gone back to normal indicating that his liver is no longer fatty. The creatinine level, which is an indicator of how well the kidneys are functioning, is essentially unchanged. This proves

Table 17. Blood Work of Mr. P Pre- and Post-Diet.				
Test	Pre-Diet	3 Months	18 Months	Normal Range
Glucose (fasting)	6.7	4.4	4.2	3.6-6.0 mmol/L
HbA1C	-	0.049	0.051	0.040-0.060
Triglycerides	2.88	0.77	0.77	<2.30 mmol/L
Total Cholesterol	6.48	5.44	4.62	5.40 mmol/L
LDL	4.09	3.67	3.01	3.40 mmol/L
HDL	1.08	1.42	1.26	0.77-1.68 mmol/L
Total / HDL Ratio	6.48	3.80	3.67	< 5
AST	54	29	18	10-40 U/L
Alkaline Phosphatase	83	66	59	40-120 U/L
GGT	75	27	-	15-73 U/L
Creatinine	99	97	85	60-125 umol/L
Micro-albumin	-	3	-	up to 30 mg/L
Albumin/ Creatinine ratio	-	0.4	-	up to 2.5
CRP	-	-	0.3	<8.0
BMI	30	26	24	<25

that this diet and the ketosis do not cause kidney damage. His urine micro albumin level and albumin to creatinine ratio is low which show that the kidneys are normal. After another calculation, he scored an 8 (decreased from 12) which gave him a 10-year risk of 4%. Due to his positive family history, we need to multiply the 4% by 2 in order to estimate his 10-year risk, which equaled to 8%. The targets for LDL cholesterol are to get below 4.5 mmol/L and the total cholesterol to HDL cholesterol ratio is to get below 6.0. This time, his blood levels were within the target limits.

Figure 7. Weight Reduction of Mr. P.

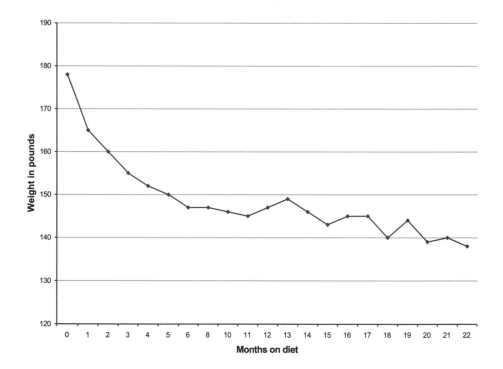

After 18 months on the diet, he is still on the Maintenance Phase and still very careful as to what he eats. Lifestyle changes are forever. Mr. P avoids things that are listed on Table 40. His weight is now 138 pounds, and his total body fat is 16% (normal is 8 to 22%). He drinks enough fluids so that his urine becomes very pale yellow color, and his percentage of total body water is 63% (normal for male is 60% to 70%).

We are sure that there are many people out there with similar story. Gains weight as they grow older. Some gains weight without causing side effect. Some gains weight and develop all kind of illnesses

It has been eight years since he started on this diet. He was able to maintain his weight following the maintenance program. If he gains some weight after vacation, he goes back to the Induction Phase for 1 week. He has successfully incorporated this diet as part of his lifestyle.

In medical school, the professors always used the term "lifestyle changes" when they talked about the management of hypertension, coronary artery disease, and diabetes. Most doctors did not understand exactly what was involved in "lifestyle changes" and doubted its effectiveness. However, we are now true believers that one can improve his health by weight loss, regular exercise, and stress reduction. We hope that we can convince our patients to do the same and change their lives for the better.

With certain susceptible individuals, obesity leads to an increase in circulating free fatty acids, which in turn causes insulin resistance. With insulin resistance, the body tries to compensate by producing more insulin, which leads to hyperinsulinemia (high level of insulin). Scientists believe that it is the combination of insulin resistance and hyperinsulinemia that produce hypertension, hypertriglyceridemia, decreased high-density lipoprotein cholesterol and hyperglycemia, which are all signs of metabolic syndrome.

In a normal individual, insulin influences bodily function through two different pathways. These two pathways have similar but opposite effects to each other, keeping everything in check and balance. For simplicity, lets call them pathway A and pathway B. Insulin acts on pathway A to produce dilatation of blood vessels, leading to a lower blood pressure. When insulin acts on pathway B, it produces vasoconstriction and water retention, which leads to a higher blood pressure. It is this check and balance that keeps your blood pressure within a narrow range. You can say that pathway A is the good pathway and pathway B is the bad one. Other bodily functions that are affected by these pathways are the growth of smooth muscle cells around blood vessels, the ability to dissolve blood clot (plasminogen activator inhibitor), the formation of plaque inside blood vessels (atherosclerosis), and inflammation.

This mechanism of check and balance breaks down when the obese patient develops insulin resistance. Insulin resistance means that the insulin produced can no longer function to its full capacity. Mainly it is pathway A that gets blocked in the insulin-resistive state. The body tries to compensate by producing extra amounts of insulin. This leads to hyperinsulinemia and over-stimulation of pathway B, and produces all kinds of bad side effects typical of Metabolic Syndrome.

In the early stages of Metabolic Syndrome, the obese patient has insulin resistance and hyperinsulinemia. The treatment is by weight reduction since it is the extra free fatty acid produced from the adipocytes that causes insulin resistance. Exercise, metformin and insulin sensitizers (Actose® and Avandia®) can also help to fight insulin resistance. The patient already has hyperinsulinemia. It dose not make sense for the doctor to prescribe insulin secretagogues such as glyburide (Diabeta®), glicazide (Diamicron®), repaglinide (GlucoNorm®), nateglinide (Starlix®) and glimepiride (Amaryl®), which induce the pancreatic beta cell to secrete extra insulin. Starting this patient on insulin at this time can also worsen the symptom of hyperinsulinemia. *Remember that insulin injections do not treat insulin resistance.* However, if the patient's diabetic control is sub-optimal due to poor eating habits and lack of exercise, the doctor has no choice but to start the patient on insulin. In this case, an insulin injection is the better of the two evils.

When the beta cells are all exhausted and no longer able to produce insulin, insulin injections will be the treatment of choice. At this stage, the patient will no longer be suffering from hyperinsulinemia. The insulin injection will merely be a replacement dose and should not be over-stimulating the B pathway.

Metabolic Syndrome occurs due to insulin resistance and hyperinsulinemia. The treatment of Metabolic Syndrome should be aimed at lowering the fat weight and the circulating insulin level. Metabolic Syndrome has become a major worldwide public health issue that warrants *early detection and intervention* in order to prevent complications.

If there is a family history of Metabolic Syndrome in first-degree relatives, and if the patient develops central obesity, we will treat the patient aggressively with dietary intervention, cognitive psychotherapy, and possibly medication. There are many ongoing trials at this time to see if certain medications can prevent or delay the development of diabetes. They are Glucophage®, Coversyl®, and Actose® just to name a few. Results are pending.

Reference:

1. Grundy SM, Cleeman JI, Daniels SR, et al. Diagnosis and management of the metabolic syndrome. An American Heart Association/National Heart, Lung, and Blood Institute Scientific Statement. Circulation 2005;112:2735-52.

6: Why did the Low Fat, Low Protein, and High Carbohydrate Diet Fail?

You have probably heard this from your friends many times:

- I work out daily and cannot lose weight

- I eat only healthy food but I gain weight

- She can eat so much and stay slim, I starve but still gain weight

- I am not eating any fat and I eat very little meat. I still cannot lose weight

We want to show you that sometimes it is *not how much* you eat, but *what* you eat that causes weight gain.

In a low-fat low-protein diet, most of your daily caloric intake will have to come from carbohydrates.

Figure 8. Fat Gain from Eating Carbohydrates.
Carbohydrate Intake = Fat Build Up

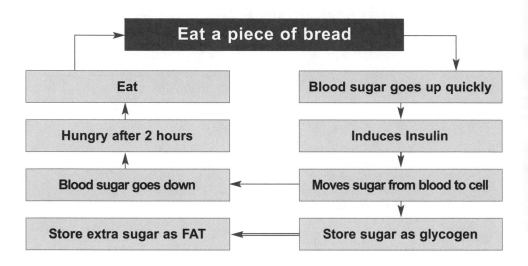

In 1996, researchers showed that subjects who followed a low-fat diet did not get rid of their obesity, did not lower their cholesterol levels, did lower their HDL levels, and increased their blood level of triglycerides level. All the above are risk factors of heart disease.

Gram for gram, fat contains more than twice the number of calories than carbohydrates (9 calories vs. 4 calories per gram). Food products that contain high amounts of fat are called "energy dense" foods. Cutting back on the amount of total fat in the diet and replacing it with carbohydrates would seem to be a great way to lose weight. It is easy to understand why experts might have first begun recommended a low-fat high-carbohydrate diet.

Cutting back on fat has not worked as well as was first hoped when it comes to weight loss. While products like low-fat crackers and non-fat cakes have crowded grocery store shelves, we have continued to get fatter and fatter. The reason is, although we are eating less fat, we are consuming even more calories than ever, and feasting on sugars and highly refined flour - otherwise known as simple carbohydrates.

Someone may say, "A calorie is a calorie. If you stay within a certain number of calories, then you will loose weight." However, research has found that a calorie from a carbohydrate is *not* the same as that from protein or fat sources. The subjects in this study were given diets with different compositions, but all added up to 1000-calories-per-day. This was considered a low calorie intake. If the calories from carbohydrates, fat and protein were the same, then you would expect all diet groups to lose the same amount of weight. The actual results showed that all diet groups resulted in different amounts of weight loss. The high carbohydrate, low fat group actually gained weight instead!

Another study done in 2003 at the Harvard School of Public Health found that consuming an extra 300 calories (20% more food) a day on a very low-carbohydrate diet resulted in more weight loss (20 pounds verses 17 pounds) than those who were on a low-fat diet over a 12-week study period. If the low carbohydrate group ate the same amount of calories as the low fat counter part, the low carbohydrate group lost 23 pounds over the same period of time. This clearly shows that 1 calorie from a carbohydrate source does not equal to 1 calorie from fat or protein. This shows that the way the body handles food that is high in carbohydrates is different from that of high protein. It will take more energy to digest 1 calorie of protein when compared to carbohydrates (thermal effect of food).

Research has shown that even when the patient stayed within the daily allowable calories, weight gain occurred in the group that had the most calories coming from carbohydrates. Papers have been written that link childhood obesity to fruit juice, sweetened juice drinks, and soft drinks. The USDA study linked high-fructose corn syrup to the development of obesity and the increase in the prevalence of Type 2 diabetes. High fructose corn syrup now represents more than 40% of sweeteners added to food and beverages. Dietary protein and fat do not require much insulin to process, whereas refined carbohydrates do. A predominantly low-fat high-carbohydrate will increase insulin levels, and it is the insulin excess that makes you fat and sick. Very low-calorie high-carbohydrate diets cause a series of chemical imbalances that make it difficult to burn stored fat and result in muscle wasting instead. Very low-calorie and low-fat diets usually cause instability of blood glucose levels, which results in fatigue and cravings that will sabotage your efforts to maintain a healthy way of eating. The body reacts to this type of diet by slowing down the body metabolism in order to save energy (decrease thyroid hormone secretion). The net effect is intolerance to cold, hair loss, and oligomenorrhea (infrequent menses). Patients may also end up with dull looking hair, skin and fingernails.

There have been *no* studies that can link a high protein diet to obesity. Some research has demonstrated that most high protein food has fat associated with it and it is the fat that causes weight gain. Also important to note is that there is no study that can demonstrate that a high protein diet can cause kidney damage in a healthy subject.

Excessive fat consumption is linked to obesity, because fat is the most calorie dense macro-nutrient as compared to carbohydrates and protein. One assumes that the total calories consumed are also high. Do not forget that the human body needs to replenish essential fatty acids daily to maintain good health. The choice of the fat source is more important than the total amount consumed (Chapter 9). The addition of some good fats to your diet can make your food taste more palatable. Fat can also provide you with the feeling of early satiety. Cholecystokinin is a peptide that is secreted from the stomach in response to fat ingestion. Cholecystokinin signals the CNS to trigger meal termination[1].

In a review paper written in 2002 looking at past data, it concluded that higher protein weight-loss diets have led to beneficial reductions in body weight, fat mass, and food intake, while preserving lean body mass and improving satiety in overweight and/or obese individuals. They also increase postprandial energy expenditure, increase fat oxidation and lower the respiratory exchange ratio[2-11].

The daily protein requirement is 0.6 g/kg of body weight. The daily requirement of essential fatty acids should be 5% of the total caloric intake. For example, for a 2000 calorie diet, there should be 6.7 g of omega-3 fatty acid (linoleic acid) and 2.2 g of omega-6 fatty acid (alpha-linolenic acid). Clinical signs of essential fatty acid and protein deficiency include alopecia, scaly dermatitis, and anemia. However, there is no daily requirement of carbohydrates. This is because the body can manufacture carbohydrates from protein and fat.

References:

1. Moran Timothy, Gut Peptide Signaling in the Controls of Food Intake. Obesity 2006;14(supp 5):250S-3S.

2. Eisenstein j, Roberts SB, Dallal G, Saltzman E. High-protein weight-loss diets: are they safe and do they work? A review of the experimental and epidemiologic data. Nutr Rev 2002;60:189-200.

3. Brehm BJ, Seeley RJ, Daniels SR, D'Alessio DA. A randomized trial comparing a very low carbohydrate diet and a calorie-restricted low fat diet on body weight and cardiovascular risk factors in healthy women. J Clin Endocrinol Metab 2003;88:1617-23.

4. Due A, Toubro S, Skov AT, Astrup A. Effect of normal-fat diets, either medium or high in protein, on body weight in overweight subjects: a randomised 1-year trial. Int J Obes Relat Metab Disord 2004;28:1283-90.

5. Layman DK, Evans E, Baum JI, et al. Dietary protein and exercise have additive effects on body composition during weight loss in adult women. J Nutr 2005;135:1903-10.

6. Leidy HJ, Carnell NS, Mattes Rd, et al. Higher protein intake preserves lean mass and satiety with weight loss in pre-obese and obese women. Obesity 2007;15:421-9.

7. Skov AR, Toubro S, Ronn B, et al. Randomized trial on protein vs carbohydrate in ad libitum fat reduced diet for the treatment of obesity. Int J Obes Relat Metab Disord 1999;23:528-36.

8. Farnsworth E, Luscombe ND, Noakes M, et al. Effect of a high-protein, energy-restricted diet on body composition, glycemic control, and lipid concentrations in overweight and obese hyperinsulinemic men and women. Am J Clin Nutr 2003;78:31-9.

9. Tannous, dit EI Khoury D, Obeid O, Azar ST, et al. Variations in postprandial ghrelin status following ingestion of high-carbohydrate, high-fat, and high-protein meals in males. Ann Nutr Metab 2006;50:260-9.

10. Bowen J, Noakes M, Clifton PM. Appetite regulatory hormone responses to various dietary proteins differ by BMI status despite similar reductions in ad libitum energy intake. J Clin Endocrinol Metab 2006;91:2913-9.

11. Johnston CS, Day CS, Swan PD. Postprandial thermogenesis is increased 100% on a high-protein, low-fat diet versus a high-carbohydrate, low-fat diet in healthy, young women. J Am Coll Nutr 2002;21:55-61.

"Lord, if you cannot make me skinny,
Please make my friend fat."

7 : Insulin is Your Enemy and Glucagon is Your Friend

You are going to learn how insulin causes obesity and stops you from utilizing fat as your energy source. It is the objective of this diet to eliminate hyperinsulinemia in order to burn fat. Insulin also increases salt and water retention (caused by excess secretion of cortisol and aldosterone), that leads to hypertension. Another way insulin causes hypertension is by its involvement in promoting the loss of magnesium. A high insulin level prevents the metabolism of triglycerides and increases your serum triglycerides level. This eventually causes arteriosclerosis. It has also been implicated in increasing the risk of Type 2 diabetes (by inducing insulin resistance), breast cancer, clotting problems, colon cancer, gout, sleep apnea, peptic ulcer disease and polycystic ovarian syndrome.

If the doctor injects insulin into your blood stream, you will experience the following effects:

1. Decreased blood glucose

2. Increased intracellular glucose level

3. Increased conversion of glucose to fat

4. Inhibited ketogenesis (burning of fat)

5. Reduced gluconeogenesis (production of glucose from other sources, e.g. amino acids and glycerol) by the liver

6. Increased storage of glycogen by liver and muscle

7. Decreased concentration of potassium and inorganic phosphate in blood

8. Decreased secretion of glucagon

The net effect will be weight *gain*. Hence, it is common to see Type 2 diabetics get fatter once they are put on insulin.

If the doctor injects glucagon into your blood stream, you will experience the following effects:

1. Increased blood glucose

2. Increased blood potassium

3. Promotes glycogenolysis (breaking down of glycogen)

4. Increased gluconeogenesis

5. Reduced motility of the gastrointestinal tract

6. Increased *ketogenesis* (fat burning)

7. Decreased secretion of insulin

The net effect will be weight *loss*.

Insulin and glucagon exert a negative feedback effect on each other. That is to say, when you have a high insulin level, your glucagon level will be suppressed, and vice versa. For weight loss purposes, you want your insulin level to be low and glucagon level to be high. Lowering the secretion of insulin is achieved by eating a low-carbohydrate diet, decreasing caloric intake, altering your dietary fat profile (eating better quality fat and decreasing the saturated fat), and increasing exercise. Westphal SA et al demonstrated that eating high levels of lean beef protein without carbohydrates evokes an extremely small rise in serum insulin levels and a concomitant substantial rise in glucagon[1].

$$\textbf{\textit{FAT}} \quad \overset{\text{Glucagon}}{\underset{\text{Insulin}}{\rightleftarrows}} \quad \textbf{\textit{BLOOD SUGAR}}$$

Most of the causes of obesity are related to hyperinsulinemia and insulin resistance.

- *Overeating.* When you overeat, particularly refined carbohydrates, the blood glucose increases. In order to maintain a normal blood sugar level, the body will have to produce and secrete more insulin from the pancreas. The more carbohydrates you consume, the higher the level of blood insulin, which eventually causes hyperinsulinemia.

- *Genetic.* A gene was identified in an experimental animal study that produces a hormone called *Leptin.* Leptin is a hormone that is secreted from the adipocytes to signal that you have enough food and to stop eating. An obese-prone individual is found to have resistance to Leptin. Therefore, this individual will overeat, leading to hyperinsulinemia. According to research, longevity can be achieved with a low calorie diet, high HDL cholesterol or genes that cause a lower serum insulin baseline level. Hence, if you develop a diet that lowers the production of circulating insulin and normal glucose, the patient should live longer.

- *Stress.* During stressful situations, either physically or mentally, your body will increase the secretion of *adrenaline* and *cortisol* as a "flight or fight" response. You will experience an increased respiration and heart rate, shakiness, sweatiness, anxiety, and dilated pupils when you are stressed. These hormones also increase your blood glucose. Hence, diabetic patients find it difficult to control their blood glucose when they are depressed or have an infection somewhere in the body. In response to the increase in blood glucose, more insulin will be secreted and this eventually causes weight gain.

- *Insulin resistance.* Due to whatever reason, either genetics or obesity, people develop insulin resistance. Their cells cannot respond to the usual amount of insulin and the pancreas has to pump out an extra amount of insulin to try to overcome this resistance. The insulin becomes less and less effective in the conversion of glucose into cellular energy, and more glucose is transformed into fatty deposits. Hence, the amount of carbohydrates that is converted into fat is much higher in people with insulin resistance as compared to normal subjects, even while consuming the same amount of carbohydrates. The more obese you are the higher degree of insulin resistance you will have and the more weight you will gain. This becomes a vicious cycle. The blood level of insulin is much higher in people with insulin resistance. Therefore, they are more prone to develop *reactive hypoglycemia* (Chapter 11). Hypoglycemia makes you tired and slows down your mental capacity. This causes a sudden urge to eat carbohydrates. If you do go and consume more carbohydrates, another *"eats and weight gain"* cycle begins. This may be the reason why obese patients always say that their friends who are thin can eat anything they want and still do not gain weight. This is because the thin individual has no insulin resistance and can process glucose more effectively.

Another hormone that may be of interest in weight control is the *Growth Hormone (Somatotrophin)*. It is a protein hormone secreted by the pituitary gland. The physiological functions of the growth hormone are:

1. Bone and cartilage growth

2. Promoting growth of organs

3. Protein anabolism (muscle growth)

4. Lipolysis (breakdown of fat)

5. Increase blood glucose (diabetogenic), free fatty acid and phosphorus

The net effect will be an increase in muscle mass and decrease in fat mass. As we grow older, the level of growth hormone drops and we increase our fat mass and decrease our muscle mass instead. It would be advantageous to increase or maintain our growth hormone level in order to stay lean. The various stimuli that have been reported to increase growth hormone secretion by the pituitary gland are:

1. Fasting

2. Low blood glucose

3. Exercise

4. High protein meal

5. Glucagon

6. Stress, mentally or physically

7. Sleep

8. Growth hormone releasing factor (from hypothalamus)

Since growth hormone is a protein compound, it will be destroyed in the gut if we take it by mouth. Growth hormone has to be given by injection or inhalation. There are herbal preparations that are supposed to stimulate the secretion of growth hormone, e.g. NGH Max Release. The efficacy has not been proven. An overdose of growth hormone in adults can lead to acromegaly.

Reference:

1. Cavadini C, Siega-Riz AM, Popkin BM. West J Med 2000;173:378-83.

8 : Ketosis

Your body stores fat when you ingest more nutrients than the body can use. When food is not readily available, your body calls on the reserves and changes the fat into usable energy. This is a normal physiological reaction for all mammals. This is particularly true in hibernating animals. During the long winter months, the bear has to utilize his fat storage to maintain his bodily functions. Hence, the bear is in ketosis while hibernating. Yet this type of ketosis never causes any ill effect to the bear.

This part of the book is written for those who are more scientifically inclined and want to know a little bit more about the biochemistry of fat metabolism. What you call fat, scientists call triglycerides. It consists of one glycerol and three long-chain fatty acid molecules.

When you break down fat, you release glycerol and fatty acids (Figure 8). Glycerol is then converted into glucose in the liver and is used up as energy. Fatty acids break down into Acetyl-Co A by a process call *beta oxidation*. Acetyl-Co A can enter into the mitochondria of the cell and go through the Kreb's Cycle and produce energy. During this process, a group of by-products called *ketone bodies* are formed. Aside from the heart, the kidney and the brain, most of the organs in our body cannot utilize ketone bodies as a source of energy. As a matter of fact, heart, kidney and brain cells can utilize ketone bodies for energy more efficiently (20%) than glucose. It is one of the wonders of nature. It is the survival of the fittest. During a famine, when food is scarce, our bodies can utilize fat as energy. Since only the heart, kidney and brain cells can utilize ketones, energy is preferentially channeled to these cells that are the most important organs that keep us alive.

One can measure the amount of ketone bodies in the blood. However, it is costly and takes time. Since these ketone bodies are eliminated via the kidney through urine, we will monitor your urine ketone level as an indirect measurement of your blood ketones, which in turn is an indirect indicator of your fat burning (lipolysis). For people who attempt this diet on their own, they can purchase Ketostix® in most neighborhood pharmacies. Most of the urine ketones come from fat metabolism, and only a small amount from amino acid metabolism. As a general rule, the higher the urine ketone concentration, the larger amount of fat you are burning. However, a negative test does not necessarily mean that you are not burning fat. You may be drinking a lot of water and your urine is so diluted that the concentration of urine ketones is too low to be detected. This is the reason we like to check the fasting urine sample, which is usually more concentrated.

There can be instances when the body composition analyzer shows that you burned fat, but negative urine ketones test using the Ketostix® . The reason is as follows. When the body burns fat, three different types of ketone bodies are formed in the blood. They are acetoacetic acid, acetone, and betahydroxybutyric acid. All three are present in the urine of patients with ketosis in relative proportions of 20% acetoacetic acid, 2% acetone, and 78% beta-hydroxybutyric acid. Ketostix® detects only acetoacetic acid and produces a false negative result if only acetone and beta-hydroxybutyric acid are present.

The presence or absence of ketones in your fasting urine sample collected on the day of you visit our office represents your body's metabolism during your sleep the previous night. This is called your *basal body metabolism* since you are not actively using your muscles while sleeping. If you can demonstrate that you are burning fat during your sleep, we are sure that you are burning fat the rest of the day because you will be much more active during the day and require the production of more energy.

If you deviated from the diet and have a high carbohydrate meal (e.g. a piece of cake), it will take three days of low carbohydrate intake before you can detect ketones in the urine again. What happens here is the glucose from your high carbohydrate meal is transformed into *glycogen* and stored in the liver and muscles. When you fast, e.g., during sleep, your body is going to call on the glycogen storage, rather than fat, as the source of fuel. This prevents you from burning fat. Your body usually has enough glycogen storage to last for 3 days. You have to use up the glycogen first before you start to burn fat and show positive urine ketones again.

Ketosis causes the urine to be more acidic; therefore, calcium is mobilized from the skeleton to buffer the urine in order to maintain acid-base homeostasis. This means that ketosis can cause osteoporosis. However, since most people are in ketosis for only a short period of time, it is unlikely that this diet will significantly contribute to an individual's overall risk for osteoporosis. If we find that you are in ketosis most of the time, we will start you on calcium and magnesium supplements. If you are having side effects from the over-production of ketones, all you have to do is introduce more carbohydrates in your diet. This is the reason why we check for ketone bodies in your urine every time you visit us.

We are trying to teach you that the production of ketones is a normal, physiological process when you lose fat weight. The amount of urine ketones is related to the amount of fat burning. Therefore, if you do not want to have too much ketosis, you have to slow down the rate of fat burning.

Some nutritional experts propose that weight loss should be achieved by eating fewer calories and increasing exercise levels to use up more calories. This means that the body has a higher energy output (by exercise) than input (eat less). Where does the extra energy come from? The experts will tell you that the energy comes from fat storage. There you go, the same end point as this diet plan, which is to burn fat. Does the eat-less-exercise-more diet produce ketones while burning fat? Of course it does. The same chemical changes with this diet when the body fat is metabolized into glucose and energy; ketone bodies are produced as by-products. It is not common to see ketone bodies in the eat-less-exercise-more diet because the rate of fat burning is slower, or because no one checks the ketones in the urine in that kind of diet. If the patient did a lot of exercise without increasing food intake, the patient will be burning fat and one can find ketones in the urine also. The bottom line is that if you do not want to have ketones in the blood or urine while dieting, the only way is to slow down the rate of fat burning! The fact that this diet can get you into ketosis means that you can get into a state of fat burning quicker and even without exercise. However, exercise will increase your rate of fat burning.

Ketosis vs. Ketoacidosis

There are *major differences between ketosis and ketoacidosis*. Even medical personnel got mixed up by these two events. Hence, you may hear from lay people and even medical professionals that this type of diet is bad for you because this type of diet promotes ketosis. They are wrong. They have mistaken ketosis for ketoacidosis.

Ketosis, as described in the beginning of this chapter, is a natural process in which body fat is converted back into usable energy to fuel the body. It is completely harmless. For early man, ketosis was the key to surviving periods of starvation. Hibernating animals, like bears, are in ketosis all winter long. Doctors have been treating children suffering from refractory seizures with a ketogenic diet. There is not yet a single scientific study to show that ketosis is harmful to a healthy person.

Ketoacidosis, on the other hand, is injurious to your body. However, it mainly happens to patients suffering from *Insulin Dependant Diabetes Mellitus (IDDM or Type 1 diabetes)*. This type of patient cannot produce his own insulin and requires daily insulin injections. If he/she forgets to take his/her insulin, or has an infection or surgery and there is an increase in the requirement of insulin, it causes an unopposed rise in the glucagon level. Glucagon increases blood glucose level by gluconeogenesis and lipolysis, which eventually leads to severe hyperglycemia (very high blood sugar). In a healthy subject, the rise in blood glucose from glucagon will stimulate the secretion of insulin and bring the blood glucose back down to the normal range. At the same time, insulin secretion will suppress the action of glucagon. With IDDM, the subject does not have much, if any, insulin reserve. Hence, the blood sugar continues to rise. The ketone bodies also rise to a level many times higher that what occurs in ordinary fasting. This leads to acidosis. Hence, the term is *ketoacidosis*. The presenting symptoms are anorexia, nausea, dehydration, and abdominal cramps. If untreated, altered consciousness or frank coma may occur.

There are home monitors that one can use to measure the capillary blood ketone level, just like the glucometer. If the patient has a glucometer level of higher than 16 mmol/L, the patient should check the blood ketones. If the blood ketone level is more than 1.5 mmol/L, the patient should seek medical attention. Urine measurement of ketone bodies is not as meaningful as blood ketone measurement. Urine testing for Acetoacetate, which rises after ketoacidosis resolves, since betahydroxybutyric acid metabolizes into acetoacetate.

In summary (Table 18), patient with ketosis that follow this low-carbohydrate low-fat diet have a normal blood glucose level and a negative urine glucose test. Patients with ketoacidosis from IDDM have blood glucose many times over the limit and always have large amounts of glucose in the urine. An increased serum glucagon level while following this diet is caused by a low blood sugar state. In patients with IDDM, it is caused by the lack of insulin. Hence, the ketosis originating from this diet is totally different from that of ketoacidosis. For people with a healthy kidney to begin with, ketosis is totally harmless and does not cause kidney damage.

Table 18. Differences Between Ketosis and Ketoacidosis.		
	Ketosis	**Ketoacidosis**
Insulin	↓	↓↓↓
Glucagon level	↑	↑↑↑
Blood Sugar	⟷ or ↓	↑↑
Urine Sugar	negative	↑↑↑↑
Urine ketone	↑	↑↑↑↑
Serum osmolarity	⟷	↑↑
Blood pH	⟷	↓↓
Dehydration	⟷ or ↑	↑↑

To a lesser degree, ketones are also formed from protein burning. During prolonged fasting, excessive exercise, and a low blood sugar state, your body will try to make glucose from burning muscle (gluconeogenesis). The building blocks of muscle protein are called *amino acids*. There are over twenty different types of amino acids found in your body. These amino acids can be found in the blood flowing to the tissues to repair any tissue damage (amino acid pool). For example, the intestines shed cells, the muscle cells get damaged, and there is hair loss every day. The liver can transform these amino acids into glucose when your blood sugar becomes low. As the amino acid pool gets depleted, muscle can metabolize its protein and release more amino acids into the blood. This can lead to muscle wasting. Hence for diets that do not allow you to eat enough protein, or if you diet by not eating, you are going to lose muscles. You need to consume good quality protein daily to maintain good health. A good protein is the type of protein that contains all the *essential amino acids* (Table 19).

Table 19. Amino Acid Pool.	
Non-essential Amino Acids	**Essential Amino Acids**
Glycine	Valine
Alanine	Leucine
Serine	Isoleucine
Cysteine	Threonine
Cystine	Methionine
Homosysteine	Phenylalanine
Tyrosine	Tryptophan
5-Htdroxytryptophan	Lysine
Thyroxine	
Aspartic acid	
Asparagine	
Glutamic acid	
Glutamine	
Arginine	
Citrulline	
Ornithine	
Hydroxylysine	
Histidine	
Proline	
4-Hydroxyproline	

We call this type of protein a *complete proteins* (e.g. meats, fish and egg). *Incomplete proteins* (e.g. protein from grains or beans) are those that do not contain all of the essential amino acids. Your body can manufacture some types of amino acids (e.g. Cysteine, Alanine, Tyrosine, etc) from other food sources, but essential amino acids cannot be synthesized by your body. You have to replace them daily. The reason we mention amino acid metabolism here in this chapter on ketosis is because during the process of transforming amino acids into glucose in the liver, some ketones are also formed. Only certain types of amino acids can form ketones and they are Isoleucine, Phenylalanine, Tyrosine, Leucine, Lysine, and Trytophan (for those who want to know). However, the majority of urine and blood ketones come form fat burning.

Figure 8. Production of Ketones from Lipolysis.

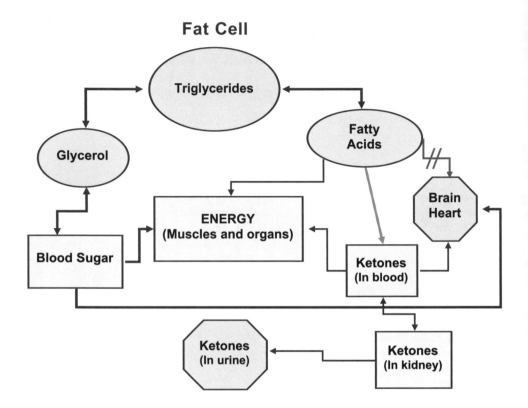

9: EAT LOW FAT AND NOT NO FAT

Fat is present in your salad dressings, seafood and cooking oil. You may use them in this diet. As a matter of fact, you need them to provide your daily requirement of essential fatty acids. Without the *essential fatty acids*, you will not be able to produce hormones and you will not be able to repair your damaged cells.

These are called *essential* because you cannot synthesize them from any other food sources other than from your daily intake. If one eats a fat-free diet, one will get sick in no time. However, we only want to eat quality fat to avoid building up unhealthy cholesterol.

The best type of fat comes from fish (high in Omega-3 oil). Use mainly olive oil or canola oil in your cooking. PAM® Cooking Spray and the Virtuous™ Cooking Spray are made from canola oil or olive oil and are suitable to use in this diet. Look for a salad dressing that is calorie-free. Do not use any creamy style dressings, e.g. Thousand Island, Ranch, or Caesar, unless they are carbohydrate-free and fat-free. Oil and vinegar is acceptable. However, rice vinegar and balsamic vinegar have higher carbohydrate content per serving (2 to 4 g) than other types of vinegar and should not be used in Phase 1 of this diet.

Avoid deep fried food and saturated fat. The oil used in repeated deep-frying might be carcinogenic (cancer causing). The chemical acrylamide is found in high levels in fried snack foods such as potato chips. The FDA also found moderate levels of acrylamide in arrowroot cookies, crackers, sweet potatoes, bottled prune juice and black olives. Omega-6 oil can be found more abundantly in sunflower, safflower and corn oils and food products made with these oils.

Do you know that your own liver manufactures about eighty percent of your blood cholesterol (using glucose and fatty acid), and only twenty percent comes from food sources? It was found that if you eat food that is rich in cholesterol; your liver would try to balance it out by producing less cholesterol. Also reported in literature was the fact that the percentage of cholesterol absorption by the intestine is decreased with an increase in dietary cholesterol content. For people who have high serum cholesterol from their dietary source, research has found that it is because there is too much saturated fat and trans fat in the diet and not due to the increase in cholesterol intake. This means that it is more important to watch the saturated fat and trans fat then to watch the dietary cholesterol level. By simply changing your diet to one that is low in starch and sugar, and high in quality fats, you can reduce elevated cholesterol, lower your triglycerides, lower the "bad" LDL cholesterol, increase your "good" HDL level, and reduce your risk for heart disease.

Most of the studies on the effect of eating fat on body cholesterol and triglycerides were done while the subjects were still eating a large amount of carbohydrates. Hence, the conclusions from these studies cannot be used to comment on this type of diet since Dr. Poon's Metabolic Diet is low in fat and carbohydrate.

A recent study has shown that a diet that is higher in fat, but lower in carbohydrates did not increase the LDL cholesterol level. The opposite is true; these patients end up with better triglycerides and HDL cholesterol levels.

Most patients and many doctors are interested mainly in the cholesterol level and do not pay much attention to the triglycerides level. High triglycerides level, irrespective of cholesterol level, is a potent risk factor for heart disease. It thickens your blood and produces arteriosclerosis.

In 1966, a Harvard researcher found that eating a low carbohydrate diet could lower the triglycerides level.

Fat ingestion has no effect on insulin induction; i.e. eating fat does not cause a rise in blood insulin level. When the fat part of your meal reaches the stomach, it triggers the secretion of the hormone *cholecystokinin*, which sends a message to your brain to say that you have enough food already and tells you to stop eating.

Another way fat helps in this diet is to slow down the absorption of carbohydrates. In other words, fat decreases the glycemic index of your carbohydrates (Chapter 11). Fat slows the rate of blood glucose increase and in turn minimizes the secretion of insulin.

Most people know that saturated fat is the "bad fat" and that polyunsaturated or monounsaturated fat is the "good fat". We now realize it is not just the polyunsaturated content of the diet, but also the ratio of Omega-6 to Omega-3 polyunsaturated fat that may ultimately determine health. The precise ratio remains controversial. The ratio should probably be in the range of 4:1. Western diets rich in cereal grains, dairy, and grain fed live stocks, drive the ratio to 10:1. This imbalance may have implications for a host of diseases, including hyperinsulinemia, arteriosclerosis and tumorgenesis.

Not only will this diet help people to lose weight, but also it is helpful in the management of a host of other common western diseases, including cardiovascular disease.

There are many types of polyunsaturated fats named under Omega-3 oil. Omega-3 means that the first double bond of this unsaturated fatty acid begins at the number 3 carbon. There are three main groups of Omega-3 fatty acids. They are alpha-linolenic acid (ALA), eicosapentaenoic acid (EPA) and docosahaexanoic acid (DHA). The most important type of fatty acid for health purposes is *docosahexaenoic acid*. It is important for the proper function of the nerve, brain and retina. The following table provides you with an idea of the content of docosahexaenoic acid in different food sources. Recommended daily intake is about 150 mg, which is not difficult to achieve.

Table 20. DHA Content of Different Kind of Fishes.	
Food	Docosahexaenoic Acid
Atlantic salmon, 3 oz cooked	1,238 mg
Rainbow trout, 3 oz cooked	697 mg
Sockeye salmon, 3 oz canned	564 mg
White tuna, 3 oz canned	535 mg
1 omega-3 egg	80 mg
3 servings of Dairy-Oh!™ milk	48 mg

Another important fatty acid is called linoleic acid (LA) which is an Omega-6 fatty acid. Only ALA and LA are considered essential fatty acids. You have to obtain them from your food sources as they cannot be produced from other macronutrients. EPA and DHA are not essential fatty acids because they can be manufactured in the body from ALA.

How often you heard that family doctors and/or dietitians recommend patients suffering from high serum cholesterol to avoid red meat and shell fish? The patients are encouraged to eat more fish instead. The reason given was that red meat and shell fish have high cholesterol levels. It is a well known fact that LDL increases the risk of coronary heart disease. However, researchers had not been able to link dietary cholesterol to coronary heart disease. Let us look at the fat and cholesterol contents in equal amounts of raw fish, lean cuts of red/white meats, and shellfish (Table 21).

Table 21. Total Fat and Cholesterol Contents of Fish, Meat and Shellfish[1].

Raw Meat Only (3 oz)	Total Fat Content	Total Cholesterol Conent
Salmon, wild sockeye	8.2	74
Cod	0.5	40
Halibut	2.0	35
Beef, sirloin	4.0	47
Pork, center loin	6.8	78
Chicken, light meat	4.0	76
Scallop[2]	0.6	28
Lobster	0.3	61
Egg, 1 large whole	4.1	212

Did you know that fish has similar cholesterol content as meat and shellfish? It was found that eating fresh fish improves a patient's cholesterol and decreases the risk of developing coronary heart disease. Obviously, it is not the dietary cholesterol that affects the patient's cholesterol. There are no studies linking egg intake (up to one egg a day) to coronary heart disease risk[3]. The daily cholesterol allowance is 300 mg. Eating a 6 oz of sirloin steak per day is well within the cholesterol limit (100 mg).

How about the fat content of food products? Research shows that it is the fat in food, particularly the saturated and trans fat, and not the dietary cholesterol that raises blood cholesterol the most. If you just look at the total fat content of a food item, then you will conclude that eating salmon is worse that eating a beef sirloin tip or chicken breast. As you break down the total fat content of the food items into saturated, monounsaturated and polyunsaturated fat, you will appreciate that although salmon is fattier than beef sirloin tip, 80.5% of the fat from salmon is the unsaturated kind. Only 47.5% of the fat from beef is the unsaturated kind (Table 22). Although different types of fish fillets have different amounts of fat, their unsaturated to total fat ratio is very similar. Lobster meat has very little amounts of fat and the unsaturated to total fat ratio is similar to that of white chicken meat. For beef and pork, the amount of fat and their compositions varies with the kind of cut chosen.

Table 22. Saturated, Monounsaturated and Polyunsaturated Fat Contents of Meat, Fish and Shellfish[1].					
Raw Meat Only (3 oz)	Total Fat (g)	Saturated fat (g)	Unsaturated (g)		Unsaturated to Total Fat Ratio
			Mono-	Poly-	
Salmon, wild sockeye	8.2	1.6	4.5	2.1	80.5
Cod	0.5	0.1	0.1	0.9	80.0
Halibut	2.0	0.4	0.8	0.8	80.0
Beef, sirloin	4.0	1.9	2.0	0.1	47.5
Pork, center loin	6.8	2.5	3.8	0.5	63.2
Chicken, light meat	4.0	1.3	1.6	1.1	67.5
Lobster	0.3	0.1	0.1	0.1	66.7
Egg, 1 large whole	4.1	1.5	1.9	0.7	63.4

Since eating fish is known to decrease the LDL and increase in the HDL levels, and lower the risk of coronary heart disease as compared to red meats, it seems to indicate that the advantage of fish is due to the good unsaturated to total fat ratio rather than the absolute amount of fat. It also indicates that it has nothing to do with the amount of dietary cholesterol present in the food. This does not mean that you can eat as much cholesterol as you wanted. Just stay within the recommended amount of 300 mg of dietary cholesterol per day. It was recommended by the American Heart Association to lower the daily intake to 200 mg per day if the patient has coronary heart disease or high cholesterol.

***Note: Some people are more prone to dietary cholesterol than other people are.

The Canada Food Guide recommended that the saturated fat should not be more that 33% of the total fat content. Except beef, all foods listed in Table 22 are within the guideline.

References:

1. USDA National Nutrient Database for Standard Reference, Release 18, Oct 2005.

2. The NutriBase Complete Book of Food Counts. Avery 2001.

3. Hu F.B. et al. A prospective study of egg consumption and risk of cardiovascular disease in men and women. J Am Med Assoc 1999;28:1387-94.

"I am on a 30 day weight loss diet, and I have already loss 16 days."

10: Medications That Can Cause Weight Gain

- *Anti-diabetic medications.* Either the injectable (insulin) or the oral form (Diabeta®, Diamicron®, GlucoNorm®, Starlix®, Amaryl®, Actos®, and Avandia®) can lead to weight gain (Table 7). These medications either directly or indirectly raise the blood insulin level. In turn insulin helps the blood glucose leave the blood stream to enter the cells (liver cell, muscle cell, etc.). Eventually the excess glucose will be stored in the adipocytes and lead to the formation of adipose tissue. The most common reason for adults to develop Type 2 diabetes is obesity. By giving obese patients this type of anti-diabetic medications, doctors are actually increasing the patient's weight. As weight increases, the body becomes more insulin resistant and requires a higher dose of medication to overcome the insulin resistance, and the vicious cycle continues. The best thing a doctor can do for this type of patient is to put him on a low-carbohydrate low-fat diet. Once the patient loses weight, the blood glucose will be under better control. The patient will require less weight gaining medication. Another commonly used anti-diabetic medication is called metformin (Glucophage®). It does not increase the production of insulin. It works by increasing the sensitivity of the insulin receptors and decreasing the production of glucose by the liver. It does not cause weight gain. Sometimes it is used to fight insulin resistance, even when the patient is not diabetic. It is also safe to use for patient who is pre-diabetic patients. Weight gain in insulin-treated patients with Type 2 diabetes was similar with different insulin regimens (except the ultra long acting insulin); the mean increase in weight at 1 year was 2.6%. In order to maintain their blood glucose, the insulin dosage keeps going up. The additional intake of metformin was associated with a 22% decrease in the required insulin dose[1].

- *Antidepressants.* Using Prozac® (Fluoxetine) and Luvox® (Fluvoxamine) as examples, they work by selectively inhibiting the neuronal re-uptake of serotonin thereby raising the serotonin level in the brain. Serotonin is a hormone that is found to be low in patients with depression. These antidepressants, by increasing the level of serotonin in the brain tissue, minimize the patient's depression. However, serotonin also acts as an *appetite stimulant* and causes the patient to overeat. Some patients refuse to go on this type of medication because they experience excessive edema and weight gain. Some antidepressants are worse than others are. Effexor® (Venlafaxine) is weight neutral but it might increase blood pressure. Celexa® (Citalopram) seems to be weight neutral. Our diet plan works well for this type of patient because the production of ketones in the body acts as a *natural appetite suppressant* and counteracts the appetite stimulating effect of serotonin. Welbutrin is weight neutral. However, it increases the risk of seizures.

- *Birth control pill and hormonal replacement therapy.* High-dose birth control pills have been associated with weight gain and water retention. The newest low-dose birth control pills are weight neutral. Implantable (Norplant®), transdermal (Estraderm®) and the injectable (Depo-Provera®) birth control medications all cause weight gain.

- *Prednisone.* This medication is used to treat arthritis, asthma, allergic reactions, and autoimmune diseases. It may cause water retention, hyperinsulinemia, increased appetite, glucose intolerance, muscle wasting, and osteoporosis if used for prolonged amount of time. It may also slow down the conversion of T_4 to T_3, which is the more biologically active form of the hormone thyroxin.

- *Nonsteroidal anti-inflammatory.* Examples are Celebrex®, Arthotec®, Mobicox®, and DayPro®. They cause water retention. That is the reason why they should not be used in a patients who are prone to congestive heart failure.

- *Beta-blocker (non-selective).* Examples will be Corgard® (Nadolol), Inderol-LA® (Propranolol), and Visken® (Pindolol). These are antihypertensive, which can block the conversion of T4 to T3. They can also cause dyslipidemia (increase serum triglycerides) and worsening of glycemic control. The newer, more selective type of beta-blocker, such as Tenormin® (Atenolol), and Lopressor® (Metoprolol) does not have this kind of side effects.

- *Calcium channel blocker.* Examples will be Cardizem® (Diltiazem), Chronovera® (Verapamil), Plendil® (Felodipine), Norvasc® (Amlodipine), and Adalat® (Nifedipine). This is a class of blood pressure medication that causes dilation of blood vessels, and in turn causes peripheral edema (swelling of the ankles).

- *Diuretics.* Examples will be HydroDiuril® (Hydrochlorothiazide), Lasix® (Furosemide), and Lozide® (Indapamide). Studies have shown that diuretics elevate blood glucose, insulin and triglycerides resulting in weight gain. It also worsens insulin resistance. This class of medication can cause hyperuricemia and gout attack. These side effects can be minimized by using a smaller dose and for a shorter period of time. Patients who take diuretics tend to drink juice or eat bananas to compensate for potassium loss. However, drinking juice and eating bananas can lead to weight gain.

- *Amiodarone.* This is a heart drug. It can cause either hyperthyroidism or hypothyroidism.

- *Schizophrenia treatment.* An example is Zyprexa® (Olanzapine). It is used in psychiatric treatment and can cause glucose intolerance and hypothyroidism that leads to weight gain. This group of patients is prone to develop Type 2 diabetes.

- *Antiseizure medications.* An example is Valproic Acid or Dilantin®. Weight gain occurs more often in females. It also causes hyperandrogenism (overproduction of male hormone) and hirsutism (increase in body hair).

- *Glucosamine sulfate.* This is used primarily in patients with arthritis of the joints. There are reports that it may cause insulin resistance.

All of these medications can make your weight loss program less effective. Even if you follow the diet plan completely, you may still have a problem in losing the desirable amount of weight. Have your doctor adjust or substitute your medications accordingly, if appropriate.

References:

1. Georg Biesenbach, Gerd Bodlaj, Herwig Pieringer. Weight gain and metabolic control in newly insulin-treated patients with type 2 diabetes with different insulin regimens. Canadian Journal of Diabetes 2006;30(4):384-9.

11: GLYCEMIC INDEX AND GLYCEMIC LOAD

Glycemic index is a term used to describe how fast the food you ingested can raise the blood glucose as compared to that of pure sugar. We assign a value of 100 as the glycemic index (GI) of pure sugar. The kind of food that has a higher GI (e.g. potato=62) will raise the blood glucose quicker than that of food with a lower GI (e.g. grapefruit=25). Food with a high GI will cause an increase in the secretion of insulin leading to weight gain. Hence, you should pick foods with a lower GI (<50). If you have two different kinds of vegetables with the same amount of absorbable carbohydrates, the one with a lower GI will be digested slower and have less impact on blood glucose. Subsequently, it will not cause hyperinsulemia; therefore, you should include this type of food in your meal plan.

For those who are interested, here is how a scientist determines the glycemic index of different food items.

- Measure the fasting blood glucose of a healthy subject.

- Give the subject 50 g of glucose solution orally.

- Measure the subject's blood glucose every 15 minutes over the next two hours.

- Plot the curve like the one on the next page.

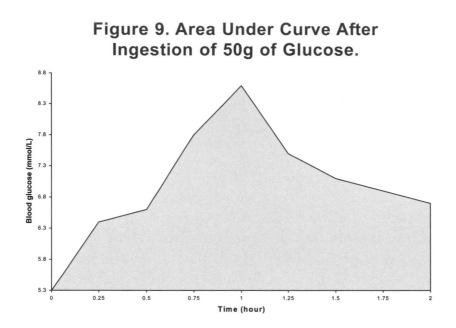

Figure 9. Area Under Curve After Ingestion of 50g of Glucose.

- Calculate the area under the curve, let say the area comes out to be "A" units.

- On the next day, the same subject has his fasting blood glucose taken.

- The subject is given an equivalent of 50 g of net-carb of the tested food item. For example, if you wish to determine the GI of spaghetti, you will give the subject 200 g of spaghetti, which contains 50 g of net-carb.

- Measure the subject's blood glucose every 15 minutes over next two hours.

- Plot the curve like the one on the next page.

- Calculate the area under the curve, let's say the area comes out to be "B" units.

- The GI of spaghetti = B/A x 100, which turns out to be 41.

Figure 10. Area Under Curve After Ingestion of 50g Net-Carb of Spaghetti.

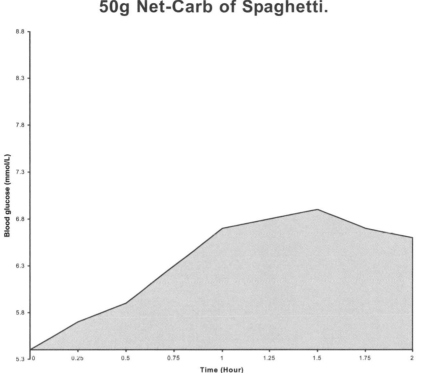

Eating food with a high glycemic index is the main cause of high serum triglycerides level, which may lead to arteriosclerosis and coronary heart disease.

A patient who consumes food with a high GI tends to develop a condition known as *reactive hypoglycemia* (low blood sugar).

With reactive hypoglycemia, the patient feels very hungry two hours after the last meal. If the patient does not eat another meal high in carbohydrates, the patient feels sweaty, shaky, headachy, lethargic, disoriented, and unable to concentrate. This is because when the patient ingests food with high glycemic values, the blood glucose shoots up sharply, which in turn triggers the release of a large amount of insulin (Figure 11, point U). The function of insulin is to drive glucose from blood into the cells, including the fat cells. However, since there is a large amount of insulin in the blood, too many glucose molecules get moved into the cells, leaving the patient with low blood glucose. The serum free fatty acid will also be low. After eating a chocolate bar the hypoglycemic symptoms go away (because the blood glucose is high now), just to come back two hours later (when his blood glucose is low, Figure 11, point D). The patient will have to eat carbohydrates to feel well again.

Figure 11. Blood Sugar After Ingestion of High Glycemic Meal.

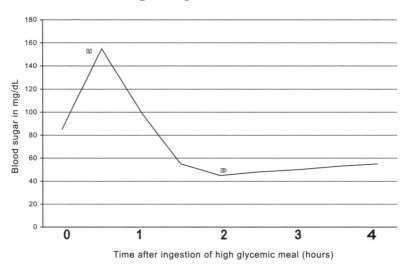

Time after ingestion of high glycemic meal (hours)

Eating foods with low GI avoids blood glucose peaks and valleys throughout the day and puts an end to mood swings and periods of lethargy. Stable blood glucose throughout the day ensures fewer food craving and false hunger pain.

This is why people who eat meals with high GI gain weight. One study shows that the size of the fat cell increases after a meal high in GI as compared to a meal low in GI, even though both have the same number of calories.

The GI of your food can be altered depending on how foods are prepared. For example, raw vegetables are more difficult to digest than cooked vegetables. It will take more time to raise your blood glucose, hence a lower GI. If you cook the pasta less tender (al dente), it is more difficult to break down the starch molecules from the pasta. The net effect is a slowing down of the digestive process. Over cooking your food also destroys more nutrients. Eating your high GI foods along with food with a low glycemic value can decrease the impact on your blood glucose. An example would be eating cantaloupe (high GI) with some ham (low GI). Two other factors can alter the GI of your meal: fat and protein. By adding fat and protein to your meal with a high GI, you will be able to lower the digestion rate of sugar and decrease the rate of blood glucose elevation. An example will be eating a slice of bread alone or eating a slice of bread with cream cheese. The rate of rise in the blood glucose is higher (higher GI) if you eat a slice of bread alone! Fat in the cream cheese slows down the digestion of the carbohydrates presented in the piece of bread. However, adding fat to the food increases the total amount of calories. Although fat can delay the rise in blood glucose, it does not dampen the total glucose response[1]. In another word, fat can slow down the absorption of carbohydrates so that the rate of increase in blood glucose after the meal is small, but with time, all of the carbohydrates ingested will be absorbed.

Refined sugar, refined flour and processed food are foods with the highest GI. You should try to avoid them. Not all low GI food is good. Fat has low GI but is not suitable for consumption. GI only applies to carbohydrates. Protein is the lowest GI food since protein consumption does not lead to blood glucose increase[1].

One of the shortcomings of GI is that it only tells us about the quality of the carbohydrates, not the quantity.

Another term commonly used is *Glycemic Load (GL)*. It describes the total amount of carbohydrate in the food ingested that can affect the blood glucose. The higher the GL, the higher the stress of the food item is on insulin and the higher chance for hyperglycemia. The GI and the total amount of net-carb presented in a particular serving size affect the value of the GL. If you eat a small bowl of lettuce, you are eating a vegetable with a low GI and can assume that it will not affect your blood glucose. However, if you eat a lot of lettuce, you are increasing the GL and can expect an adverse effect on your blood glucose. The GL is more important than GI for this diet plan.

	Glycemic Index	Glycemic Load
Table 20. Different Levels of Glycemic Index and Glycemic Load.		
Low	< 50	< 10
Medium	50-70	10-20
High	> 70	> 20

Using strawberry and prunes as an example. As shown in the Appendix, the GI of strawberries is 40 whereas the GI of prunes is 29. This means that both strawberries and prunes have low GI (Table 20). Prunes even have a lower value than strawberries meaning that the rate of increase in blood glucose is slower for prunes than strawberries. However, when the GL is calculated, you will see a big reversal. The way to calculate the GL is to take the GI and multiply it with the net-carb, and then divide it by 100.

For ½ cup of strawberries, there is a total of 4 g of net-carb (see Appendix).

GL of ½ cup of strawberries = 40 x 4 / 100 = 1.6 (low)

GL of 1 cup of strawberries = 40 x 8 / 100 = 3.2 (low)

For ½ cup of prunes, there is a total of 46 g of net-carb.

GL of ½ cup of prunes = 29 x 46 / 100 = 13.3 (medium)

GL of 1 cup of prunes = 29 x 92 / 100 = 26.6 (high)

Since the GL of ½ cup of strawberries is very low, it is safe to be included in this diet while following Phase 2. Even if you over-eat and have the whole cup, the GL is still within the safe zone. However, eating ½ cup of prunes can induce stress to the insulin; eating the whole cup will be detrimental to the diet and patient's glycemic control.

Here are a few more examples of fruit and juice that are disallowed in this diet.

GL of 1 banana = 55 x 32 / 100 = 17.6

GL of 5 dried dates = 103 x 27 / 100 = 27.7

GL of 1 cup of orange juice = 46 x 26 / 100 = 12

GL of 1 cup of spaghetti = 41 x 52 / 100 = 21.3

Even if the GI of spaghetti is low, it is not good for the diet since the GL is high. For this diet, the food items should be low in both GI and GL. You can lower the GL by simply eating smaller portions. If you eat only ½ cup instead of 1 cup of spaghetti, the GL will drop from 21.3 to 11.6.

Use the glycemic index and glycemic load values as a guideline only. The way the food is prepared and the interaction with other food items affect these values.

Although a GL of less than 10 is considered as low, this diet will only allow food items that have a GL of less than 3 because this is a low-carb diet (see appendix).

Reference:

1. Peters AL, Davidson MB. Protein and fat effects on glucose responses and insulin requirements in subjects with insulin-dependent diabetes mellitus. Am J Clin Nutr 1993;58:555-60.

12: Reading Food Labels

Food is comprised of three types of macronutrients: protein (e.g. egg white), fat (e.g. lard), and carbohydrates (sugar) (Figure 12).

Figure 12. Three Types of Macronutrients.

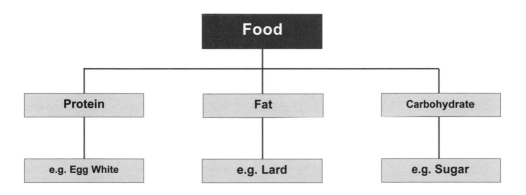

The above examples are very clear cut and people can separate them out easily. However, when you shop in the supermarkets, the food products are not as clear-cut. They are usually a combination of all three macronutrients. For example, is peanut butter a protein, a fat, a carbohydrate, or all of the above? Patient will often tell us that peanut butter is considered as a protein. Let us look at the nutritional information of a store-brought peanut butter. Out of one tablespoon of this product, 3.1 g are protein, 7.5 g are fat, and 2.9 g are carbohydrates. If we convert it to calories, 12 calories come from protein, 68 calories come from fat, and 12 calories come from carbohydrate. Either way, fat is the predominant component. Since this diet allows only minimal amounts of fat and carbohydrates, peanut butter will not be a product that you should consume. The objective of this chapter is to teach you to identify good verses bad products for this diet plan. This book is not to teach you about eating "healthy". You can learn to eating healthy food from the Canada Food Guide for Healthy Eating.

Advertisers will do every trick in the book to make you buy their products. That is their job. They may not necessarily lie but they will *bend* the truth. Things like "no added sugar" can mean that there is a lot of sugar in the food already and means that they did not add *any more* sugar, or *honey* was added instead. Things like "low fat" can be full of carbohydrates. Things like "light" can be low in fat and calories, but high in carbohydrates. Things like "low-calorie" or "low-sugar" does not necessarily mean low carbohydrate.

Table 21. Understanding the Claims on Labels.	
Writen As	**What It Actually Means**
Calorie-free	< 5 cal per serving
Calorie-reduced	25% fewer cal of the original product
Low-calorie	< 40 cal per serving
Low in sugar	< 2 g of sugar per serving
No sugar added	Contains naturally present sugar
Unsweetened	Contains naturally present sugar
Sugar-free	< 0.5 g of sugar per serving
Sugar-reduced	25% less sugar per serving
Cholesterol-free	< 2 mg of cholesterol per serving
Low cholesterol	< 20 mg of cholesterol per serving
Fat-free	< 0.5 g per serving
Fat-reduced	25 % less fat per serving

Writen As	What It Actually Means
Low-fat	< 3 g of fat per serving
Low-saturated fat	< 2 g of fat per 100g, < 15% of cal
Lean per serving	< 10 g fat, < 4.5 g sat fat, < 95 mg cholesterol
Extra lean	< 5 g fat, < 2 g sat fat, < 95 mg cholesterol per serving
Lean ground beef	maximum 17% fat content
Regular ground beef	maximum 30% fat content
Sodium-free (salt-free)	< 5 mg per serving
Low-sodium	< 140 mg of sodium per serving
Very low sodium	< 35 mg per serving
Light in sodium	Reduced by 50%
Imitation product	Less protein or less nutrients than the original
Light	If 50% or more of the calories are from fat, fat must be reduced by at least 50%per serving. If less than 50% of the calories from fat, fat must be reduced at least 50% or calories reduced by 1/3 per serving. "Light meal" can mean either "Low Calories"or "Low Fat"
Total Fat	Weight of all individual fatty acid plus weight of one unit of glycerol for each three fatty acids
Total Carbohydrate	Total weight of the food sample minus the weight of crude protein, total fat, moisture, and ash
Sugars	Total weight of all monosaccharides and disaccharides
Low-Carb	No standard yet
Source of fiber	2 g or more fiber per serving
High fiber	4 g or more fiber per serving

There is no definition of "low-carb" at this time. It can mean "low net-carb" which means it can have a lot of carbohydrates but the portion that affects the blood sugar is low. These low carb products can contain a lot of sugar alcohol that carries some calories. There is no actual number attached to the word "low-carb". It can be one gram of net-carb, or it can be 10 grams of net-carb. "Low-carb" can also mean "low absorbable carb" which means total carbohydrate minus the fiber (non-absorbable carbohydrate) and sugar alcohols (partial absorbable carbohydrate). Then the amount of "absorbable carbohydrate" will equal to the sum of sugar and starch. However, how low is low? There is no definition.

Hence, you have to learn how to read the nutritional information and the ingredients written on the labels. Do not rely on the information advertised to the front part of the label. The data on the nutritional information label is certified by the laboratory and approved by the government. Here is a label copied from a Tomato with Beef Ravioli Soup can. The total volume of the can is 540 ml.

NUTRITION INFORMATION

Per 250 ml Serving

Energy	133 Cal/560 kj
Protein	4.5 g
Fat	1.2 g
Carbohydrate	26 g
Dietary Fibre	3.3 g
Sodium	925 mg
Potassium	311 mg

First of all, since the information is per 250 ml serving, there are two servings in one can of soup. If you eat the whole can, you need to double the numbers written on this label.

Let's look at one serving only. The listed carbohydrate (26 g) on the label is actually the total carbohydrate (absorbable and non-absorbable). The dietary fiber (3.3 g) actually equals to the non-absorbable carbohydrate, which means that this is the type of carbohydrate you cannot digest or absorb.

Total Carbohydrate - Non-absorbable Carbohydrate = Absorbable Carbohydrate
        (26 g)   (3.3 g)   (22.7 g)

For your diet purposes, only the 22.7 g of absorbable carbohydrate counts. This is because only 22.7 g instead of the 26 g of carbohydrate listed on the label will get absorbed and affect your blood sugar and weight. If you eat the whole can, you will be taking in 45.4 g of carbohydrates.

Not all companies list the amount of dietary fiber on their products. However, you can read the labels of similar products from different companies and the numbers should be very similar. Another thing that you should pay attention to is the type of fat in the product. Here is a label copied from a New England Clam Chowder Ready-To-Serve Soup can. The total volume of the can is 540 ml.

NUTRITION INFORMATION
Per 250 ml Serving

Energy	195 Cal/820 kj
Protein	5.5 g
Total Fat	8.1 g
(37% Calories from Fat)	
Polyunsaturate	0.2 g
Monounsaturates	2.3 g
Saturates	3.9 g
Cholesterol	17 mg
Total Carbohydrates	25 g
Sugar	2.4 g
Starch	19 g
Dietary Fibre	1.3 g

Again, there are two servings per can. Double the numbers if you eat the whole can. For any diet, you want to avoid the intake of *saturated fat*. As shown in the label above, the type of fat in this soup is comprised mainly of the saturated kind. Hence, it is not good for your health (see Table 24).

Reading the number of calories per serving may be necessary if you are over eating and require calorie counting. The daily allowable calories that you can have are shown in Table 39.

Read the ingredients on the label. Avoid the products that have white flour, cornstarch, corn syrup, sugar, dextrose, maltose, lactose, honey, salt and hydrogenated vegetable oils as the main ingredients. They list the ingredients according to the weight. The ingredient with the highest weight percentage will get listed first. Hence, if an ingredient is listed as the eighteenth ingredient, it is not likely to have a big impact on the nutritional value.

Another term you may encounter frequently in diet food products is *Net Effective Carbohydrates (Net-carb)*. This is a label copied from a package of sugar free Gummy Bears. It said "0 sugar carb" in the front.

NUTRITION INFORMATION

Serving size: 17 pieces

Calories	100 cal
Calories from Fat	0 cal
Total Fat	0 g
Saturated Fat	0 g
Cholesterol	0 mg
Sodium	5 mg
Total Carbohydrate	30 g
Dietary Fiber	0 g
Sugar	0 g
Sugar Alcohol	30 g
Protein	3 g

Since our body does not absorb sugar alcohol effectively, although the total carbohydrate is 30 g, the Net Effective Carbohydrate is 0 g (read Chapter 20). This means that the amount of carbohydrate that can increase the blood glucose is zero. However, a net effective carbohydrate of 0 does not mean that there are no calories. The 3 g of protein contribute 12 calories (3 g x 4 calories per g). Hence there are 88 calories (100 - 12) contributed by the sugar alcohol. Because there is no fiber in this product (no non-absorbable carbohydrate), the total amount of absorbable and partially absorbable carbohydrate is still 30 g.

Caution. A few years ago, when the low-fat diet was popular, people only looked at the fat and cholesterol contents. No one cared to watch the amount of carbohydrate intake and people got fatter. The food industry took pride in advertising their products as low in fat or cholesterol free. Today, people are so fixated on the low-carbohydrate diet and care about the carbohydrate content only and they forget to look at the fat and cholesterol contents. The newer food products are all advertised as low-carb. Read the whole label and not just one part of it. Remember that this is a low-sodium, low-carbohydrate *and* low-fat diet. Food items should conform to all three criteria before it is considered suitable for this diet.

The American Heart Association recommends the total intake of fat to be less than 30% of your total calorie intake. The amount of saturated fat should be less than 10% of the total calorie intake. This diet program would like to see you eat as little saturated fat as possible.

Our diet program will let you know what your daily metabolic rate is supposed to be according to your age, sex, weight and height using a body composition analyzer. You can then figure out your maximum daily allowance of total fat and saturated fat intake using Table 22. Remember that these values apply only to healthy subjects. Patients with diabetes or high serum cholesterol should limit their saturated fat to the bare minimum. There is no health benefit in ingesting cholesterol, as your body (liver) can manufacture cholesterol from other sources. Although the allowable daily cholesterol is around 300 mg, we feel the daily requirement of cholesterol should be zero. However, eating a small amount of cholesterol in the diet will not increase your LDL cholesterol and it will not increase your coronary heart disease risk.

Table 22. Maximum Daily Allowance of Total Fat and Saturated Fat.		
Daily Calories	Max. Grams of Total Fat	Max. Grams of Saturated Fat
1,200	40	13
1,400	47	16
1,600	53	18
1,800	60	20
2,000	67	22
2,200	73	24
2,400	80	27
2,600	87	29
2,800	93	31
3,000	100	33

This is a label copied form a bag of Milk Chocolate Covered Almonds. It also said "0 sugar carb" in the front part of the packaging.

Nutrition Information

Serving size: 10 pieces

Calories	210 cal
Calories From Fat	150 cal
Total Fat	17 g
Saturated Fat	7 g
Total Carbohydrate	18 g
Dietary Fiber	2 g
Sugars	0 g
Sugar Alcohol	16 g
Protein	4 g

If you just look at the Net Effective Carbohydrate count, both the Gummy Bears and Milk Chocolate Almond products are the same (0 g). However, there are two major differences between these products that make the Gummy Bears suitable for this diet and not the Milk Chocolate Almonds. The Milk Chocolate Almonds have more than double the calories per serving. It also contains a high amount of fat and saturated fat. The calories from fat (153 calories) accounts for 70% of the total calories (should be less than 30%). Out of the 17 g of total fat, 41% is saturated fat (should be less than 33%).

Here is another example of how manufacturers advertise their products in order to mislead the consumers into buying their products. This is written on the front of a package of Sugar-free Brown Rice Cake - "0 sugar". On the backside of the package, you will find the nutrition facts.

Nutrition Information

Serving size: 1	
Total Fat	9 g
Saturated Fat	5 g
Cholesterol	4 mg
Sodium	10 mg
Potassium	12 mg
Total Carbohydrate 25 g	
Fiber	1 g
Sugars	0 g
Maltitol	14 g
Protein	2 g

Ingredients: Maltitol, whole grain brown rice, cocoa butter, chocolate liquor, calcium carbonate, dairy oil, calcium caseinate, flaxseed oil, soya lecithin, salt, vanilla.

They also advertised it as "A Sugar-Free Low Glycemic Snack". However, is it a low carbohydrate product? They did not lie about the sugar content that was zero. "No sugar" does not mean that it is carbohydrate free. When you add up the weight of fiber, sugars and Maltitol (see Chapter 20), it comes to 15 g. However, as listed on the label, the total carbohydrate value is 25 g. Ten grams of carbohydrates are not listed on the label. This 10 g of carbohydrates likely comes from the "whole grain brown rice" in the form of starch. A more appropriate label would be "a Sugar-Free High Carbohydrate Snack". Because starch from brown rice has a lower glycemic index than simple sugar, they advertised it as a "Low Glycemic Snack". The effective carbohydrate is 10 g, which can still raise the blood sugar and trigger an insulin response.

What you should do when you look at a food label, is not to just look at a few selected items. If you just concern yourself about sugar, you may miss the other kinds of absorbable carbohydrates. Look at the serving size, the amount of calories per serving, the amount and types of fat, the amount of effective carbohydrate, and the amount of sodium. Glance at the first few items listed on the ingredients to get a feeling as to what you are about to eat. There is no need to count the protein and fiber since there is no limit of these two items in this diet plan. Keep in mind that you should have over 25 g of fiber intake per day.

The following table shows you the recommendations issued by the U.S. Food and Drug Administration (USDA) Center for Food Safety and Applied Nutrition in regarding to reference values for nutrition labeling in a diet based on a 2000 calorie intake. This gives you an idea as to what a "healthy" diet is supposed to look like for healthy adults and children 4 or more years of age. However, a healthy diet does not necessarily mean that it can help you to lose weight of help you to fight disease. For example, if you have high blood pressure, the 2400 mg of sodium intake per day will be too high for you.

Table 23. Reference Values for Nutrition Labeling, Based on a 2000 Calorie Intake; for Adults and Children 4 or more Years of Age.

Nutrients	Daily Values
Total Fat	65 g
Saturated fatty acids	20 g
Cholesterol	300 mg
Sodium	2400 mg
Potassium	3500 mg
Total carbohydrate	300 g
Fiber	25 g
Protein	50 g
Vitamin A	5000 IU
Vitamin C	60 mg
Calcium	1000 mg
Iron	18 mg
Vitamin D	400 IU
Vitamin E	30 IU
Vitamin K	80 g
Thiamin	1.5 mg
Riboflavin	1.7 mg
Niacin	20 mg
Vitamin B	2 mg
Folate	400 g
Vitamin B12	6 g
Biotin	300 g
Pantothenic acid	10 mg
Iodine	150 g
Magnesium	400 mg
Zinc	15 mg
Selenium	70 g
Copper	2 mg
Manganese	2 mg
Chromium	120 g
Molybdenum	75 g
Chloride	3400 mg

(USDA Center for Food Safety and Applied Nutrition April 2008).

A patient asks me if he can eat a product that contains only 10% sodium. I usually answer him with a question. What does 10% sodium mean to you? Using the following label as example, it is a can of octopus in garlic flavoring.

NUTRITION FACTS

Amount/serving		%DV
Total Fat	4 g	6%
Saturated Fat	1 g	5%
Trans Fat	0 g	
Cholesterol	40 mg	13%
Sodium	240 mg	10%
Total Carb	3 g	1%
Protein	14 g	

%DV stands for percent daily values. Using table 23, the daily intake allowance for sodium is 2400 mg. Since there is 240 mg of sodium in one serving of this octopus, it represents 10% of the daily allowance of sodium intake. In order to make the 10%DV of sodium become meaningful; you will need to know your daily allowance for that specific nutrient, in this case 2400 mg of sodium. On the other hand, we look at the actual quantity per serving, in this case 240 mg, which is slightly higher than what is allowed in a low-sodium diet (see table 24).

Dr. Poon's Metabolic Diet promotes food products that are low in sodium, low in carbohydrates *and* low in saturated and trans fats. A perfect meal will be one that contains a good quality and quantity of protein, some poly- or mono-saturated fat, is high in fiber, low in simple carbohydrates, cholesterol and saturated fat, sodium free and low in calories. Any food product that deviates from these rules may not be suitable for our diet. Table 24 shows you some guidelines when you try to decide which food products are desirable and which ones to avoid. The product should not have more than 1 g of net carb (for Phase 1), and less than 10 g of sugar alcohol per serving. Less than 30% of the total calories should come from fat. The maximum amount of total fat is 6 g. Out of this 6 g, there should be less than 2 g (33%) of saturated fat. The cholesterol and sodium content should be as low as possible.

Table 24. Ingredients of a Good Food Product (per serving)

- < 1 g of net-carb (sugar + starch + maltodextrin) for Phase 1
- < 5 g of net-carb (sugar + starch + maltodextrin) for Phase 2
- < 10 g of net-carb (sugar + starch + maltodextrin) for Phase 3
- < 10 g of sugar alcohol
- < 30 g of polydextrose + inulin
- < 30% of calories coming from fat
- < 6 g of total fat
- < 2 g of saturated fat (total fat : saturated fat > 3 : 1)
- < 30 mg of cholesterol
- < 170 mg of sodium
- No limit on protein and fiber

Here are the labels of some of the products that may of interest to you. You decide if they are good for your diet. We have written some hints at the end of the product descriptions to help you to identify the potential problems that can arise if you are not careful.

The ingredient list on a food label is the listing of each ingredient in descending order of predominance by weight. The ingredient that weighs the most is listed first, and the ingredient that weighs the least is listed last.

BELGIAN SUGARLESS TREATS, MARSHMALLOWS

Serving size:1 (7.5 g)	
Calories:	15.3 cal
Carbohydrates total:	5.82 g
Sugar alcohol:	5.76 g
Net-carb:	0.06 g
Fat:	0 g
Proteins	0.375 g
Sodium:	0.05 g

Ingredients: Water, sweeteners (Isomalt, maltitol, maltitol syrup, and lactitol), gelatin, natural colors and natural flavoring (vanilla)

Hint: We allow you to have two servings at a time, why? How much sugar alcohol do we allow you to have per serving?

Muffin Mix, Chocolate Chip

Serving size: 1 muffin (28 g)

Calories: 100 cal (mixture), 190 cal (prepared)

Total fat:	1 g
Saturated fat:	0 g
Cholesterol:	0 mg
Sodium:	210 mg
Total carbohydrate:	12 g
Dietary fiber:	5 g
Sugar:	0 g
Sugar alcohol:	5 g
Protein:	11 g

Ingredients: Soy protein, maltitol, chocolate drops, whey protein, gluten flour, inulin, erythritol, corn fiber, guar gum, natural and artificial flavors, polydextrose, cream, lecithin, baking powder, xanthan gum, sodium aluminum phosphate, salt, sucralose, acesulfame potassium.

Hint: High calorie prepared. The calorie and fat content of the dry muffin mix is not bad. It increases after you add eggs and oil to bake the muffin.

Cereal Bars, Cinnamon Bun

Serving size: 1 bar (36 g)

Calories:	100 cal
Total fat:	2.7 g
Saturated fat:	1.3 g
Trans fat:	0 g
Cholesterol:	4.5 mg
Sodium:	94 g
Total carbohydrate:	22 g
Dietary fiber:	2 g
Sugars:	0 g
Sugar alcohol:	17 g
Protein:	2.7 g

Ingredients: Cinnamon bun filling (maltitol, sorbitol, water, modified tapioca starch, natural flavor, glycerine, pectin, locust bean gum, cinnamon, red#40, blue#1), maltitol syrup, corn starch, palm shortening (non-hydrogenated palm oil, isomalt, whey protein concentrate, enriched bleached wheat flour (niacin, reduced iron, thiamine mononitrate, riboflavin, folic acid), polydextrose, wheat protein concentrate, isolated soy protein, vegetable glycerine, wheat bran flour, powdered cellulose (high fiber source), salt, baking soda, mono- and diglycerides, soy lecithin, vegetable gum (carrageenan, sodium chloride), natural flavors, monocalcium phosphate, sucralose.

Hint: Look at the Total fat to Saturated fat ratio. Look at the amount of sugar alcohol. You should consume one half of a bar at a time. You can eat the other half after 4 to 5 hours.

PANCAKE & WAFFLE MIX

Serving size: 1 pancake (approx. 16 g)

Calories:	63 cal
Total fat:	1 g
Saturated fat:	0.6 g
Cholesterol:	32 mg
Sodium:	136 mg
Total carbohydrate:	5 g
Dietary fiber:	2 g
Polydextrose:	1.4 g
Sugars:	0 g
Protein:	8 g

Ingredients: Ultrafiltered whey protein concentrate, soy protein isolate, whole eggs, polydextrose, whole cream, soy fiber, guar gum, monocalcium phosphate, sodium bicarbonate, natural buttermilk flavor, sucralose.

Hint: You still have to add other ingredients, e.g. egg and milk when you prepare the pancake. Net-carb in the dry mix is 1.6 g, higher after preparation. Can you just eat 1 pancake?

TANGERINE-GRAPEFRUIT FLAVORED DIET DRINK MIX

Serving size: 250 ml/2 g

Calories:	4 cal
Protein:	0.1 g
Fat:	0 g
Carbohydrate:	0.3 g
Aspartame:	59 mg
Acesulfame-potassium:	15 mg

Ingredients: Citric acid, calcium fumarate, natural and artificial flavor, color, aspartame, sodium citrate, magnesium oxide, acesulfame-potassium.

Hint: Fat and carb free, minimal amount of sodium.

Jell-O-Light™, Tropical Twists

Serving size: ½ cup (125 ml)

Calories:	7 cal
Protein:	1.3 g
Fat:	0 g
Carbohydrate:	0 g
Aspartame:	43 mg
Acesulfame-potassium:	14 mg

Ingredients: Gelatin, adipic acid, sodium citrate, sodium phosphate, artificial flavor, aspartame, salt, acesulfame-potassium, color.

Hint: Fat and carb-free, but has no sodium listed in the ingredients.

Breyers® Creamsicle™

Serving size: 50 ml

Calories:	20 cal
Protein:	1.0 g
Fat:	0 g
Cholesterol:	0 g
Carbohydrate:	6 g
Sugar:	g
Polydextrose:	3.8 g
Aspartame:	33 mg

Ingredients: Milk ingredients, malto-dextrin, polydextrose, glycerine, mono- and diglycerides, pectin, guar gum, aspartame, locust bean gum, polysorbate 80, artificial flavor. Water ice: polydextrose, cellulose gel, citric acid, guar gum, carrageenan, aspartame, natural and artificial flavor, color.

Hint: Fat-free, net-carb low (2.2 g), sugar alcohol low..

BREYERS® FAT FREE FUDGSICLE™

Serving size: 50 ml

Calories:	40 cal
Protein:	3 g
Fat:	0.2 g
Cholesterol:	2.7 mg
Carbohydrate:	10 g
Sugar:	2 g
Polydextrose:	3.9 g
Aspartame:	41 mg

Ingredients: Milk ingredients, polydextrose, maltodextrin, modified milk ingredients, cocoa, cellulose gel, powdered malt, aspartame, mono- and diglycerides, cellulose gum, salt, carrageenan, locust bean gum, artificial flavor, polysorbate 80.

Hint: Higher calorie than Creamsicles™, net-carb is higher also (6 g).

CHAPMAN'S NO SUGAR WATER ICE TREATS

Serving size: 1 lolly (50 ml)

Calories:	27 cal
Protein:	0 g
Fat:	0 g
Carbohydrate:	7.7 g
Sugars:	0 g
Maltitol:	4.0 g
Sorbitol:	0.2 g
Sucralose:	8 mg

Ingredients: Water, maltitol, maltodextrin, citric acid, sorbitol, guar gum, sucralose, natural and artificial flavor, color.

Hint: What is the net-carb? This is very tricky. The answer: net-carb equals to 3.5 g. Although it did not list the quantity of starch, when you read the ingredient list of this product, you cannot locate anything that is made from starch. However, when you look at the ingredients, you see maltodextrin. It is not a sugar but it is a polymer of simple sugar molecules. Its glycemic index is just like dextrose (glucose), which is very high. Since maltodextrin is listed as the third ingredient on the list, its weight has to be somewhere between 0.2 g (sorbitol) and 4.0 g (maltitol). Subtracting the weight of sorbitol (0.2 g) and maltitol (4.0 g) from the total carbohydrates (7.7 g) will give you the weight of maltodextrin, which is equal to 3.5 g. Hence, the net carb is 3.5 g.

DIET MERINGUES, VANILLA

Serving size: 3 pieces (4.5 g)

Calories:	12 cal
Total fat:	0 g
Cholesterol:	0g
Sodium:	5 mg
Total carbohydrate:	4 g
Sugars:	0 g
Sugar alcohol:	4 g
Protein: 0.5	g

Ingredients: Modified malt egg whites, natural and artificial vanilla flavor, xanthan gum, salt, vinegar, sucralose.

Hint: Sugar alcohol. Maximum 2.5 servings at a time.

TOFU CHOCOLATE FUDGE TREATS

Serving size: 1 piece (40 g)

Calories:	30 cal
Total fat:	0 g
Cholesterol:	0 g
Sodium:	86 mg
Total carbohydrate:	6 g
Dietary fiber:	0 g
Sugars:	0 g
Sugar alcohols:	4 g
Protein:	1 g
Lactose:	0 g
Potassium:	61 mg

Ingredients: water, maltodextrin, sorbitol, polydextrose, cocoa processed with alkali, soy protein, tofu, mono and diglycerides, cellulose gum, carrageenan, vanilla with other natural flavors, aspartame, salt.

Hint: Fat-free, net-carb = 2 g.

DIET COUNTRY SPICE HOT CEREAL

Serving size: 40 g (1/2 cup)

Calories:	170 cal
Total fat:	7 g
Saturated fat	0.5 g
Cholesterol:	0 g
Sodium:	130 mg
Total carbohydrate:	15 g
Dietary fiber:	12 g
Sugars:	0 g
Protein:	12 g

Ingredients: Wheat bran, soy protein concentrate, flaxseed meal, pumpkinseed flour, spices, salt.

Hint: High fat (but they are the good kind) and calories. Net-carb of 3 g.

Are there really 170 calories in ½ cup of this cereal? There are 9 calories per gram of fat and 4 calories per gram of protein and carbohydrate. Nine calories per gram multiplied by 7 grams of fat equals to 63 calories. Four calories per gram multiplied by 15 grams of carbohydrates equals to 60 calories. Four calories per gram multiplied by 12 grams of protein equals to 48 calories. The total calorie count is 63 plus 60 plus 48 that equals to 171 calories.

However, there is one problem with the calorie count derived from carbohydrates. The total carbohydrate is 15 and the amount of fiber is 12 grams, hence the amount of starch is 3 grams. Therefore, 12 calories come from the 3 grams of starch. The other 48 calories come from the fiber. However, since human cannot digest fiber, the actual calories added to our diet is much lower than 48. So why do the manufacturers include the calories from fiber into the total calorie count? It is because of the law. Canadian law states that *all* carbohydrates have to be included in the final calorie count even if we cannot digest them. It can pose a problem for people who try to lose weight using the calorie counting method. The same product, if sold in USA, will have a calorie count of 122 on the label. It is because the labeling law in US is different. They consider all fiber to have zero calories.

DELICIOUS PROTEIN SHAKE WITH THERMOGEN-X

Serving size: 1 scoop (15.5 g)

Calories:	60 cal
Protein:	12 g
Total fat:	0.5 g
Saturated fat:	0 g
Cholesterol:	5 mg
Total carbohydrate:	1 g
Sugars:	0 g
Dietary fiber:	0.5 g
Sodium:	100 mg
Potassium:	168 mg

Ingredients: Soy protein isolate, whey protein concentrate, whey protein isolate, natural strawberry flavor, xanthan gum, cellulose gum, carageenan, guarana seed extract, silica, sobitol, stevia leaf, bromelain, papain, amylase, glucoamylase, protease, acid protease, cellulose, lipase, kola nut, lecithin, white willow bark, meadowsweet herb, wintergreen, green tea extract, xylitol, flaxseed powder, citrus aurantium extract, salicin extract, red beet powder.

Hint: Low-fat low-carb low-sodium high-protein.

CREAMY VANILLA SHAKE

Serving size: 1 can (325 ml)

Calories:	170 cal
Total fat:	9 g
Saturated fat:	1.5 g
Cholesterol:	15 mg
Sodium:	170 mg
Potassium:	580 mg
Total Carbohydrate:	4 g
Dietary fiber:	3 g
Sugars:	1 g
Protein:	20 g

Ingredients: Water, calcium caseinate, soybean oil, whey protein concentrate, cellulose gel, natural and artificial flavors, potassium phosphate, cellulose gum, soy lecithin, Carrageenan, sucralose, beta carotene, magnesium chloride, magnesium phosphate, tricalcium phosphate, D-biotin, D-calcium pantothenate, folic acid, niacinamide, pyridoxine hydrochloride, sodium ascorbate, thiamin mononitrate, and other vitamins and minerals.

Hint: Low-carb high-fat product.

SMOKED CHICKEN BREAST ROAST DELI

Serving size: 100 g

Calories:	98 cal
Protein:	18 g
Fat:	2 g
Carbohydrate:	2 g
Sodium:	1240 mg
Potassium:	360 mg

Ingredients: Chicken breast, water, salt, glucose solids, sodium phosphate, carrageenan, dextrose, sodium erythorbate, sodium nitrite.

Hint: How much sodium should you have in a day? How much sodium should you have per serving?

Fat Free Chicken Breast 35% Less Sodium

Serving size: 100 g

Calories:	103 cal
Protein:	18 g
Fat:	0.7 g
Polyunsaturated:	0.2 g
Monounsaturated:	0.3 g
Saturated:	0.2 g
Cholesterol:	30 mg
Carbohydrate:	6.1 g
Sodium:	559 mg
Potassium:	762 mg

Ingredients: Chicken, water, corn syrup solids, potassium chloride, salt, flavor (modified corn starch), yeast extract, sodium phosphate, carrageenan, sodium erythorbate, sodium nitrite.

Hint: How much salt are you allowing per day and per serving?

All Beef Wieners

Serving size: 1 wiener (75 g)

Calories:	200 cal
Fat:	16 g
Saturated:	6 g
Trans fat:	0.1 g
Cholesterol:	15 mg
Sodium:	750 mg
Carbohydrate:	6 g
Fiber:	0 g
Sugars:	2 g
Protien:	8 g

Ingredients: Beef, water, modified corn starch, modified milk ingredients, salt, sugar, sodium erythorbate, sodium nitrate, spice, flavor (garlic), smoke.

Hint: Where does the fat come from? How much fat per serving is allowed? Out of the 16 g of fat, what is the maximum amount of saturated fat allowed? Salty! Net-carb of 6 g.

DELI-SLICED ZESTY GARLIC PICKLES

Serving size: 2 slices (28 g)

Calories:	4 cal
Protein:	0.1 g
Fat:	0 g
Carbohydrate:	0.8 g
Sugar:	0.5 g
Starch:	0 g
Fiber:	0.3 g
Sodium:	220 mg
Potassium:	28 g

Ingredients: Cucumbers, water, white vinegar, salt, dehydrated garlic and peppers, spices, seasoning, calcium chloride, turmeric.

Hint: Very low calories. Watch the salt.

SEASONING BLEND

Serving size:	0.7 g
Calories:	2 cal
Protein:	0.1 g
Fat:	0.1 g
Carbohydrate:	0.5 g
Sodium:	1 mg
Potassium:	10 mg

Ingredients: Onion, spices, herbs, garlic, orange peel, tomato, lemon juice solids, citric acid, oil of lemon.

Hint: Low in everything.

Mayo Ultra Low Fat

Serving size: 1 tablespoon (15 ml)

Calories:	17 cal
Protein:	0 g
Fat:	0.4 g
Polyunsaturated:	0.2 g
Monounsaturated:	0.1 g
Saturated:	0.1 g
Cholesterol:	2 mg
Carbohydrate:	2.8 g

Ingredients: Water, sugar, modified corn starch, vinegar, soybean oil, salt, egg yolk, citric acid, pectin, xanthan gum, modified milk ingredients, color, lactic acid, potassium sorbate, mustard, calcium chloride, calcium disodium EDTA, spices and seasonings, dried garlic.

Hint: Not good for Phase 1 but ok for Phase 2. It is low in fat but the net-carb is too high for Phase1.

Italian Vinaigrette Dressing

Serving size: 15 ml (1 tablespoon)

Calories:	36 cal
Protein:	0 g
Fat:	4 g
Carbohydrate:	0.1 g
Sucralose:	1 mg

Ingredients: Water, soybean oil, white and red wine vinegar, salt, dried garlic and red bell pepper, spices, xanthan gum, monosodium glutamate, natural flavor, sorbic acid, sucralose and sulphites.

Hint: Higher fat as compared with other light dressings.

Italian Dressing

Serving size: 15 ml (1 tablespoon)

Calories:	6 cal
Protein:	0.4 g
Fat:	0.2
Polyunsaturated:	0.2 g
Monounsaturated:	0.1 g
Saturated:	0.1 g
Cholesterol:	0 g
Carbohydrate:	0.8 g

Ingredients: Water, vinegar, sugar, soybean oil, garlic puree, salt dried garlic, xanthan gum, dried onion, dried red bell pepper, black pepper, red pepper, oregano, tarragon, calcium disodium EDTA, color.

Hint: Good product but the sodium content not listed.

Diet Steak Sauce

Serving size: 1 tablespoon (15 ml)

Calories:	6 cal
Protein:	0.1 g
Fat:	0.1 g
Carbohydrate:	1.1 g
Sucralose:	0.9 g

Ingredients: Water, Tomato paste, vinegar, salt, raisin paste, Worcestershire sauce, modified corn starch, orange juice concentrate, natural flavor, fried garlic and onion, spices, color, soybean oil, xanthan gum, sodium benzoate, potassium sorbate, citric acid, sucralose.

Hint: No sodium content listed. However, you can get this kind of information by calling or writing to the company directly. It contains 195 mg of sodium per serving. Is it too high?

Canadian Sardines in Tomato Sauce

Serving size: 106 g (1 can)

Calories:	136 cal
Protein:	17 g
Fat:	6.3 g
Polyunsaturated:	2.2 g
Polyunsaturated Omega-6:	0.4 g
Polyunsaturated Omega-3:	1.1 g
Monounsaturated:	2.6 g
Saturates:	1.3 g
Cholesterol:	92 mg
Carbohydrate:	2.5 g
Sodium:	520 mg
Potassium:	262 mg

Ingredients: Sardines, water, tomato paste, modified cornstarch, salt, sugar, soya oil, citric acid, xanthan gum, polysorbate 80, spices.

Hint: Most canned food has too much salt (sodium).

Smoked Sockeye Salmon

Serving size: 57 g

Calories:	104 cal
Total fat:	4.9 g
Saturated fat:	1.2 g
Cholesterol:	15 mg
Sodium:	421 mg
Total carbohydrate:	0 g
Protein:	15 g

Ingredients: Sockeye salmon, natural alder smoke, salt.

Hint: Watch the salt.

Chunk Light Tuna in Water

Serving size: 60 g

Calories:	65 cal
Protein:	15 g
Total Fat:	0.6 g
Polyunsaturated:	0.3 g
Monounsaturated:	0.1 g
Saturated:	0.2 g
Cholesterol:	30 g
Carbohydrate:	0 g
Sodium:	199 mg
Potassium:	129 mg

Ingredients: Tuna, water, salt.

Hint: Watch the salt. It is more appropriate to call this "Chunk Light Tuna in Salty Water". Sixty gram serving size equals to half of a can.

Frozen Whole Leaf Spinach

Serving size: 100 g

Calories:	31 cal
Protein:	2.9 g
Total fat:	0.3 g
Total carbohydrate:	4 g
Sugars:	0 g
Starch:	1.0 g
Dietary Fiber:	3 g
Sodium:	74 g
Potassium:	323 mg

Ingredients: Spinach.

Hint: Good source of fiber.

Fresh Cut™ Whole Leaf Spinach (canned)

Serving size: 125 ml

Calories:	34 cal
Protein:	3.3 g
Fat:	0.6 g
Carbohydrate:	4 g
Sodium:	490 g
Potassium:	400 g

Ingredients: Spinach, water, salt.

Hint: Watch the salt. Canned food has more salt than the frozen counterpart.

Quick Oats

Serving size: 30 g

Calories:	117 cal
Protein:	4.2 g
Fat:	2.1 g
Polyunsaturated:	0.8 g
Monounsaturated:	0.7 g
Saturates:	0.4 g
Cholesterol:	0 g
Carbohydrate:	20 g
Fiber: 2.2 g	

Ingredients: 100% Prairie grown oats.

Hint: Are Oats classified as protein, fat, or carbohydrate? How much is starch?

Fibre Cereal

Serving size: 30 g (1/2 cup)

Calories:	110 cal
Fat:	1 g
Saturated:	0 g
Trans fat:	0 g
Cholesterol:	0 g
Sodium:	130 mg
Carbohydrate:	24 g
Fiber:	15 g
Sugar:	0 g
Protein:	2 g

Ingredients: Wheat bran, corn bran, corn starch, maltodextrin, natural color, guar gum, calcium carbonate, sodium carboxymethylcellulose, salt, sodium bicarbonate, corn oil, aspartame, sulphites.

Hint: Good source of fiber. What is the net-carb? Can you eat this in Phase 1?

Part-Skim Mozzarella 18% m.f.

Serving size: 30 g

Calories:	86 cal
Protein:	7.7 g
Fat:	5.4 g
Carbohydrate:	0.6 g

Ingredients: Partially skimmed milk, modified milk ingredients, bacterial culture, salt, enzyme, calcium chloride.

Hint: Low-carb high-fat.

Ultra Low Fat Cream Cheese product 4% m.f.

Serving size: 15 g (1 tablespoon)

Calories:	18 cal
Protein:	1.6 g
Fat:	0.7 g
Carbohydrate:	1.5 g

Ingredients: Milk ingredients, light cream cheese, water, modified milk ingredients, cornstarch, maltodextrin, salt, lactic acid, natural flavor, carob bean gum, mono and di-glycerides, sodium citrate, potassium sorbate, calcium propionate, sorbic acid.

Hint: Much lower in fat and calories than cheese.

Large Egg

Serving size: 1 large egg (50 g)

Calories:	75 cal
Protein:	6 g
Fat:	5 g
Omega-6 polyunsaturated fat:	0.8 g
Omega-3 polyunsaturated fat:	0.05 g
Monounsaturated fat:	1.9 g
Saturated fat:	1.6 g
Cholesterol:	216 mg
Carbohydrate:	0.5 g

Hint: High cholesterol. Daily allowance is 300 mg.

Liquid Egg Product

Serving size: 50 ml (50 g)

Calories:	49 cal
Protein:	5 g
Fat:	2.5 g
Omega-6 polyunsaturated fat:	0.3 g
Omega-3 polyunsaturated fat:	0.4 g
Monounsaturated fat:	1 g
Saturated fat:	0.8 g
Cholesterol:	42 mg
Carbohydrate:	0.6 g

Ingredients: Liquid egg white, liquid whole egg, Menhaden oil, soy lecithin, beta carotene, xanthan gum, citric acid, natural flavor, alpha tocopherol.

Hint: lower in calories, cholesterol, fat and saturated fat. Ratio of Omega-3 to Omega-6 is better.

Canned Chicken broth 25% less sodium

Serving size: 125 ml

Calories:	13 cal
Protein:	2.5 g
Fat:	0.1 g
Carbohydrate:	0.6 g
Fiber:	0.1 g
Sodium:	610 mg
Potassium:	352 mg

Ingredients: Chicken broth, salt, yeast extract and hydrolyzed wheat gluten, chicken flavor, dextrose, potassium chloride, disodium guanylate, disodium inosinate, spice, ascorbic/citric acid blend, caramel and beta carotene.

Hint: The regular chicken broth contains 990 mg of sodium per serving. The daily sodium intake for patients with high blood pressure or water retention should not be more than 1200 mg per day.

DIET WHEAT BREAD

Serving size: 1 slice (28 g)

Calories:	60 g
Fat:	1 g
Saturated fat:	0.2 g
Trans fat:	0 g
Cholesterol:	0 mg
Sodium:	130 mg
Carbohydrate:	7 g
Fiber:	1 g
Sugar:	0 g
Protein:	5 g

Ingredients: Water, whole wheat flour, wheat gluten, soybean flour, yeast, sugar, vegetable oil, salt, vinegar, mono and/or diglycerides, calcium propionate, acetylated tartaric acid esters of mono and diglycerides, ammonium chloride, calcium iodate, sorbic acid.

Hint: Net-carb of 6 g. Lower in calories.

100% WHOLE WHEAT BREAD

Serving: 1 Slice (27 g)

Calories:	70 cal
Fat:	1.5 g
Saturated fat:	0.2 g
Trans fat:	0 g
Cholesterol:	0 mg
Sodium:	140 mg
Carbohydrate:	9g
Fiber:	3 g
Sugars:	0 g
Protein:	5 g

Ingredients: Water, whole wheat flour, wheat gluten, wheat protein isolate, oat hull fiber, vegetable oil, slat, vinegar, sorbic acid, calcium propionate, calcium sulphate, sodium stearoyl-2-lactylate, monoglycerides, malt extract, sucralose.

Hint: The net-carb is 6 g.

13 : EXERCISES

Multiple clinical trials were done to find out the effectiveness of diet only, exercise only, and a combination of diet and exercise in the treatment of obesity. The most weight loss came from the diet and exercise group. Exercise is also found to be extremely important in the success of the maintenance program. The current recommendation is a total of 150 minutes of exercise per week (e.g. 30 minutes of walking five times per week).

Even if the patient exercises daily, they still may not be able to lose any weight, because most patients eat the wrong types of food after they exercise and replenish the calories and glycogen burned during the exercise. During exercise, the obese patient uses the glycogen stored in the muscle and liver as the main source of fuel. One of my patients is a chef in a health club. He told me that, very often, club members work out for an hour and then come out to the café and order beer and pizza. If the patient eats a meal high in carbohydrates, the glycogen that was burned during exercise will reform. Even if the patient works out the next day, only the newly formed glycogen will be used instead of the stored fat. The stored fat was never touched. It is the body fat that you need to lose and not just body weight. Exercise without the right diet will not burn fat, unless you exercise many hours a day. Most obese patients have very poor exercise tolerance. It would be unreasonable to expect them to do hours of exercise per day. Hence, this diet does not require patients to do exercise in the Induction Phase. This does not mean that you should stop exercise. Just continue with your routine. When the patient is burning fat by demonstrating a positive urine ketones test, then we will start the patient on an exercise program. At that time, the source of fuel used during exercise will be coming from *fat* since the glycogen storage in muscle and liver has been depleted during the Induction Phase.

The benefit of exercise does not just stop at weight reduction. It was found that increased physical activity reduces insulin resistance and improves glucose tolerance in the diabetic patient. Exercise was found to prevent the development of hypertension, and increase the level of HDL cholesterol.

There are two general types of exercises that you need to do, and both are important for your diet program. However, it is more important that you begin with the diet first before starting to exercise. People who exercise but eat the wrong type of food will *not* lose weight.

Table 25. Amounts of Exercise (in minutes) that You Need to do in Order to Burn-off the Calories from Your Food.		
Food	**Walking**	**Cycling**
Apple	19	12
Raw Carrots	8	5
Pizza	35	22
Beer	19	12
* Do not expect to lose weight if you have a slice of pizza and a bottle of beer after 30 minutes of exercise.		

SOURCE: J. AM. DIETITIC ASSOC. (1965), 46:186, KONISHI, F.

Cardiovascular Exercises

Walking, jogging, aerobics, and dancing all involve deep breathing. The heart rate goes up and the body uses up energy (calories). Although this diet does not require you to count calories, the lower your calorie intake, the more fat you can burn. However, just by lowering the calories in your diet is not a very effective way to lose weight. Even if you decrease your intake by 500 calories per day, you can only lose 1 pound per week. These types of exercises improve your endurance, flexibility and muscle strength. They also help to lower your insulin production and resistance, improve your mood, decrease body pain (by the production of Endorphins), and elevate the good cholesterol (HDL) and bone density. Aerobic exercise helps with depression. The maximum benefit of exercise is achieved when you reach your Target Heart Rate (THR). To find your THR, subtract your age from 220, than multiply it by 0.7. For example, if your age is 48, you subtract 48 from 220, which equals to 172. Multiply 172 by 0.7, which equals to 120. Your goal is to do your cardiovascular exercises until your heart rate reaches 120 beats per minute. However, this may not be achieved overnight. You should start with a low impact type of exercise and try to increase your heart rate to 75% that of your THR; i.e. 90 beats per minute. As your endurance improves, increase your exercise time and the degree of difficulty gradually until your THR is reached. Patients who have coronary heart disease, hypertension, stroke, diabetes, or dizzy spells should consult their doctor to arrange an exercise stress test before doing vigorous exercises.

Lifestyle changes such as using the stairs instead of using the elevator, parking farther away in the parking lot or walking to the corner store instead of using the car can be helpful. Health benefits associated with physical activity, including a healthy body weight, are more closely related to the intensity rather than duration of physical activity.

Here are a few pointers about walking and jogging.

- Wear the right type of clothing and shoes

- Relax your muscles, especially the muscles in the shoulders

- Bend your elbows at 90 with your palms facing downward

- Do not make fists

- Swing your upper extremities in the same direction as your walking. Do not swing your upper extremities from side to side. Do not swing your hand higher than your heart

- Take deep breaths using your abdomen and your rib cage

- Do not bounce up and down. Keep your head still

- Put your center of gravity a little bit forward

- Lead with your knees when you run

Muscle Building Exercises

These exercises do not burn as many calories. However, by increasing your lean body mass, you increase the number of calories your body naturally spends just to keep functioning. This is the way to increase your body metabolism. Muscle is your fat burning engine. The bigger the muscle mass, the bigger the engine and the more fat will be burned away. It also helps you to reshape your body.

All organs require a constant amount of energy to function properly. For our daily energy expenditure, 20% is used up by the muscle, 17% by the liver, 10% each by the bowels, brain and heart, 6% by the kidneys and 4% by the lungs. Since the size of your liver, bowels, brain, heart, kidneys and lungs are fixed, only the muscle mass can be increased significantly to increase your metabolic rate.

There are two different kinds of muscle fibers. The type 1 fiber is a slow fiber with a high oxidative rate. It has large amount of mitochondria and uses fat as the main source of energy. You can increase the number of type 1 fibers through endurance exercises. If you can increase the amount of mitochondria in this type of fiber, more fat can be burned. The number of mitochondria can be increased by weight reduction. The type 2 fiber is a fast fiber and utilizes glucose and glycogen as the source of energy. It contains only a small amount of mitochondria. The number of type 2 fibers can be increased with muscle strengthening exercises.

To avoid injury, do not use dumbbells that are too heavy. The right weight will be the amount that will cause fatigue at five to eight repetitions. If you do not wish to build muscle, do fifteen to twenty repetitions to tone your muscles. Once you can do more than ten repetitions of muscle building exercises, increase the resistance. A program for general fitness or strength should typically include all the major muscle groups of the body and exercise muscles around each joint (neck, shoulders, upper back, lower back, abdominal, front and back of upper leg, calf, front and back of upper arm, front and back of forearm).

There are three types of muscle contractions during the muscle building exercises. They are *ISOMETRIC, DYNAMIC CONCENTRIC*, and *DYNAMIC ECCENTRIC*. During an isometric contraction, the muscle contracts but no movement takes place, as when you hold a book in front of you without letting the book drop to the ground. It is not unusual to have a patient who has back, hip, and knee problems that limit the patient's ability to exercise. Isometric exercise is a good way to exercise the big muscles without aggravating the sore joints. With the patient sitting on a chair, keep the back straight. Raise one leg in full extension and hold it horizontal to the ground as long as you can. You should feel the thigh muscle tightening up. Let your leg come down slowly and repeat with the other leg.

A dynamic concentric contraction takes place when the muscle contracts and shortens and movement occurs. For example, a dynamic concentric contraction of the biceps occurs when you flex the elbow while lifting a free weight. A dynamic eccentric contraction takes place when the muscle contracts and lengthens and movement occurs. Lowering a free weight from the flexed elbow position is a dynamic eccentric contraction of the biceps. Using all three types of muscle contractions is superior to using only one type of movement. Hence, during your weight lifting exercises, pay attention to both the concentric and eccentric phases. Let the weight down slowly rather than dropping the weight using gravity.

Proper breathing technique is important. You should *inhale* just before and during the lowering phase of the repetition and *exhale* during the lifting phase. With isometric training, you should not hold the breath during a muscular contraction. When you hold your breath, blood pressure rises drastically. This makes it very difficult for the heart to pump blood and reduces blood return to the heart. When you exhale, blood flow to the head and brain is reduced. This can cause light-headedness. This is why you want to exhale during the lift and inhale during the lowering phase.

Obesity makes it difficult to take deep breaths. In order to take a deep breath, the chest wall has to expand and move outward, and the diaphragm has to contract and move downward. Central obesity or intra-abdominal obesity causes an increase in the intra-abdominal pressure and the diaphragm has difficulty in moving downward. Chest wall expansion is also limited by the presence of extra fat on the chest. One way to compensate for the inability to inhale fully is to make sure that you fully exhale. If you can get rid of as much air as possible from your lungs, the total amount of fresh air that can move into your lungs will be increased. One such technique is to squeeze your navel inward as if you want to touch the spine with your navel while exhaling through your mouth. As you let go of the navel quickly, inhale though your nostrils. You should feel a rush of air going into the lungs.

Research has found that weight gain is related to stress. People tend to overeat when they are stressed. Junk foods are their food of choice. Exercise helps to relieve stress by releasing a hormone called Endorphin. This is why people feel good after exercise.

Again, if you have high blood pressure and/or coronary heart disease, consult the doctor before doing high-energy exercises.

Patient on long term corticosteroid treatments may experience lower muscle mass. Using Growth hormones or testosterone to counteract the catabolic effect of corticosteroid was not successful. Exercise is the only solution to maintain the muscle mass and to limit fat gain.

Sit-ups

The basic sit-up is a popular way of working your abdominal muscles. Start off by lying on your back with your knees bent, making sure your feet are flat on the floor. Do not do sit-ups with straight legs. It may hurt your back. Do not anchor your feet.

Bring your feet in towards your bottom and place your hands and arms according to your abdominal strength. The closer your hands are to your head, the more difficult sit-ups become. As a beginner, rest your hands at your side. As you get stronger, you can cross your arms across your chest. Eventually, cross your arms behind your head. Do not interlace your fingers at the back of head. This may injure your neck. Try to keep your eyes on the ceiling even when you pull forward.

Bring the shoulders and upper body up towards your knees in a slow even pace. Do not jerk up quickly. Exhale while you go up. Come up to

213

an angle of no more than 45 degrees. There is no need to go further than this. As you go up further, you will be using the hip muscles instead of the abdominal. It is actually easier to do sit-ups when you go all the way up to the sitting position. Try to keep your chin off your chest and keep your elbows out by your side. After you reach the 45-degree angle, hold the position for two seconds and than slowly curl down. Inhale at this time. Do not let your head touch the floor when you come down. Keep the abdominal muscles tense. This part of the exercise is just as important as the first part. Repeat the whole sequence again.

If you find that sit-ups are too demanding, try doing only the curl-down phase. Assume a sitting position by pushing yourself upward with your arms. Slowly lower to the floor, keeping your abdominal muscles tensed.

This exercise will only tone your abdominal muscles. It will not burn off your fat around the abdomen by itself. You need to diet as well.

How much exercise should you do? A simple answer is the more the better. It does not matter if you do 45 minutes in one sitting or three 15 minutes short bouts. It seems that the total amount of time spent determines the total amount of weight loss.

Strenuous, unaccustomed eccentric exercise leads to muscle damage. Symptoms include delayed-onset muscle soreness (24 hours), presence of intramuscular proteins in the blood (CK), and prolonged decrements in muscle function as evidenced by reductions in strength, power output and range of motion. They are substantially reduced after a second bout of unaccustomed eccentric exercise, referred to "the repeated-bout effect". This means that you will be able to tolerate your exercise routine more easily if you persisted.

The body has to spend energy to repair the damaged muscle. Hence the actual amount of calories used during exercise is the sum of the calories burned during exercise and the calories used up for tissue repair. It is more effective than simply take in fewer calories.

You can find more exercise routines in our recipe and exercise book.

"Any amount of exercise is better than no exercise"

14: Vitamins and Nutritional Supplements

If you were grossly overweight before you started on this diet, you should have plenty of nutrients stored inside your body. Hence, you do not have to worry about supplementation during the Induction Phase. This diet has all the necessary vitamins and minerals when done correctly. Routine supplementation is not necessary. However, if you have certain medical conditions, it may be advisable to take supplementation as necessary. We are going to deal with supplements that relate to this weight loss program only.

- *Multivitamin.* Taking a daily over the counter multivitamin should not hurt you. There are four kinds of fat-soluble vitamins and you should be careful since overdosing them can be risky. They are vitamin A, D, E and K. Taking too much of these four vitamins can cause liver damage. People who are on Coumadin® (blood thinner) should not take extra vitamin K. Vitamin K will increase you Coumadin® requirement, and you should repeat your blood test to check your international normalized ratio (INR). Vitamin E, (400 IU per day) is a powerful antioxidant and may prevent cell damage caused by oxidation. Some claim that it is an anti-cancer and anti-aging vitamin. Doses of Vitamin E should not exceed the 400 IU per day limit. In higher doses, it may augment the effect of Coumadin® and cause bleeding. Long-term use of high doses of Vitamin E may also increase the risk of death by all causes. Studies suggest that circulating concentrations of vitamin D may be inversely related to the prevalence of diabetes, blood glucose concentrations, and to insulin resistance. A daily dosage of 10,000 IU of vitamin D in healthy adult was shown to be safe. However, the U.S. Dietary Reference Intake Tolerable Upper Intake Level of Vitamin D for children and adult was set at 2000 IU per day. Fish is a good source of vitamin D.

- *Vitamin B 12, Vitamin B 6, and Folic acid.* These are good for the elderly who have a problem absorbing these nutrients. The malabsorption is made worse by taking gastric acid lowering medication (e.g. Losec®, Pantoloc®, and Zantac®). The presenting symptoms will be tiredness, fatigue, anemia, and depression. Sometimes we have to give patients a *vitamin B12 injection* to fix this problem. Some commercial diet programs require the clients to stay on a very low calorie diet and they require a vitamin injection routinely. The vitamin injection itself does not help you to lose weight. These vitamins have been shown to lower the blood *homocysteine* level. High homocysteine levels were found to cause heart disease by damaging the lining of the blood vessels, leading to atherosclerotic plaque. Its level was found to be high in 25% of patients with heart disease. However, the role of homocysteine as an independent risk factor for coronary heart disease has been subject to many debates, since several studies have not found this association to be independent of other risk factors. It has also been suggested that elevation of plasma homocysteine is a consequence and not a cause of atherosclerosis. Patients taking metformin may require vitamin B12 and folate supplementation because their absorption in the intestine can be affected[1].

- *Chromium picolinate 200mcg to 400mcg* may have some positive effect on weight loss. It helps to increase muscle mass, decrease body fat and lower cholesterol. A cell study conducted by scientists at the Pennington Biomedical Research Centre in Baton Rough, Louisiana, showed that chromium picolinate increases the amount of AMP-activated protein kinase in skeletal muscle cells, thus improving insulin function and insulin sensitivity.

- *L-carnitine 1000mg and Co-enzyme Q10 60mg* are supposed to help with fat metabolism. They are also powerful anti-oxidants. Meat is the major source of carnitine. In general, the redder the meat, the higher the carnitine content is. Co-enzyme Q10 is present in both meats and vegetables. If you have difficulty in losing weight even if you are eating the right foods, you may want to try these supplements. Both have no known major side effects. These supplements are quite pricey. Patients with a high cholesterol level will very often be taking a medication in the "statin" group, such as Lipitor®, Lescol®, Pravachol®, Zocor®, Crestor®, and Mevacor®. This group of medications causes a drop of Co-enzyme Q10 and potentially decreases your ability to metabolize fat. It has been reported that a decrease in myocardial ubiquinone (Co-enzyme Q10) level could lead to impaired cardiac function in patients with borderline congestive heart failure. It is a good idea to take this supplement if you are taking any of the above statin medications. If your urine demonstrates ketones in the dipstick test, then you are able to metabolize fat and you therefore have no need to take these supplements. Taking Co-enzyme Q10 supplements daily might help to prevent some of the side effects of statin medications such as muscle aches.

- *Calcium 500mg to 1000mg* is very important for the postmenopausal female. You can take it alone or with Magnesium, or with vitamin D. This diet is low in calcium in Phase 1 since the amount of diary product is limited. Some calcium is lost via the kidney when the body goes into ketosis. However, there are other sources of food other than diary products to provide your daily calcium requirement. One cup of whole milk contains 244 mg of calcium. The amount of calcium that is present in a block of tofu is 360 mg, one large cucumber with the peel is 301 mg, 1 piece of halibut fillet is 320 mg, one cup of frozen spinach is 291 mg, one cup of fortified soymilk is 245 mg, and one cup of strawberries is 166 mg. Did you know that one ounce of cheese only provides 28 mg of calcium? Do not use TUMS as your calcium sources because it has some carbohydrates. Calcium supplementation is known to decrease visceral fat and not total body fat.

- *Magnesium 300 to 600mg* helps to regulate calcium metabolism. Hyperinsulinemia causes magnesium deficiency that can lead to heart disease, hypertension, diabetes, asthma or chronic bronchitis, chronic fatigue syndrome, migraine headaches, muscle cramps, premenstrual syndrome, anxiety, depression and other psychiatric disorders. Magnesium intake is associated with lower fasting insulin concentrations among women. Hence, it is useful in women suffering from polycystic ovarian syndrome. The RDA for magnesium is 320 mg for women and 420 mg for men. Magnesium is involved in some of the enzymes that regulate glucose metabolism. It is also a co-factor in the signal transduction action pathway of insulin. You can buy a preparation that has a combination of *Calcium, Magnesium, and vitamin D all in one pill (Jamieson™)* and take it once or twice a day, or take 3 capsules of our Metabolic Diet Supplement per day.

- *Potassium.* Potassium supplements, like Slow-K, K-Dur, Micro-K, and Kaochlor require a doctor's prescription. There are potassium preparations in lower doses that you can buy over the counter, such as Swiss Natural Sources™, No Salt™, or Salt Substitute™ that you can buy in the supermarket. Because you will be drinking at least 8 glasses of water a day and ketones act as a diuretic, you may lose a lot of potassium in the urine. A low serum potassium level may cause muscle weakness, cramps, and an irregular heartbeat. Whether you need to take a potassium supplement depends on the blood results. Do not use juice or bananas as your source of potassium, even if you are taking diuretics, because they are high in sugar. Potassium supplementation may be contraindicated for patients with renal failure.

- *Garlic.* Helps to fight cholesterol and some believe that it boosts your immunity. Different companies make garlic pills with different concentrations. Follow the instructions on the label.

- *Flaxseed oil or Omega 3-6-9 oil or fish liver oil.* They help you to improve your good cholesterol levels (HDL). Omega-fatty acids can be found in abundance in fish and grain products. Note that while Omega 3-6-9 and fish liver oil contain cholesterol, flaxseed oil does not. There is evidence that the omega-3 fatty acids in fish improve brain function in middle-aged people and actually lower the risk of mental impairment as people age. Ideally, the high-risk group should consume 40-60 g of fish per day[1]. Patients should take this type of supplement if they do not eat seafood.

- *Niacin*: Niacin is very effective in lowering the triglycerides and increasing the good cholesterol (HDL). Niacin reduces the clearance of HDL, hence increasing the HDL level. There are a few side effects with this vitamin that limit its usefulness in treating dyslipidemia. In order to be effective, a high dose of niacin is needed. However, it causes high blood glucose if one uses more than 3 g per day. Hence, one should use less than 1.5 g per day. There are two types of niacin preparations readily available now - intermediate acting and long acting. The intermediate acting niacin preparation is taken three times per day. This preparation gives people hot flashes and some people actually go to the emergency room thinking that they are having a stroke. The long acting preparation has less of this side effect and only requires taking it once a day. The drawback is that this preparation can be hepatotoxic (causing liver damage). The newest version is an extended release preparation that has no effect on diabetes and hepatotoxicity. Hot flushes are still a problem. It also requires periodic liver enzyme surveillance.

- *Conjugated linoleic acid (CLA).* Conjugated linoleic acid is a fatty acid found in beef, dairy products and seeds. The industry claims that 3 to 5 g of CLA supplementation daily can build lean muscle, burn fat, and act as an antioxidant. It might also possess anti-cancer properties. However, one of the drawbacks of CLA is that it can worsen diabetic control.

- *Doctor Poon's Metabolic Diet Formula.* There are a total of 10 ingredients in each capsule. They are niacin, vitamin B6, vitamin B12, vitamin D, folic acid, calcium carbonate, chromium picolinate, CoQ10, magnesium chelate and potassium chloride. It is formulated to help with fat burning, improve your lipid profile, blood pressure and glycemic control. It should never be used as a substitute to our diet program. There is no magic bullet. This supplement should be taken two to three times per day.

- *Diet pills.* It is very important to understand that diet pills are the last resort and not the first. It is to be used for short term, and not for more than 3 months. Do not rely on pills to lose weight. Three commonly used diet pills in Canada are Ionamine® (phenteramine), Meridia® (sibutamine) and Xenical® (orlistat). Ionamine® is an appetite suppressant. The usual dosage is 15 to 30 mg daily at noon. Since it is a CNS stimulant, it can cause hypertension, insomnia, palpitations and tremors. The worst side effect is primary pulmonary hypertension that can be fatal. Meridia® works by enhancing of satiety and increasing of energy expenditure by induction of thermogenesis. It is contraindicated in patients with a history of coronary heart disease, uncontrolled hypertension, congestive heart disease and an irregular heart beat. Do not take Meridia® together with MAIO. The usual dosage is 10 to 15 mg daily at noon. Xenical® works by binding to lipase in the stomach and intestine. This inhibits the digestion of triglycerides into fatty acids and glycerol, hence limiting the absorption of fat from the food ingested. The usual dosage is 150 mg three times per day. The undigested fat will be excreted out along with the fecal matters. Too much fat in the diet will lead to greasy diarrhea. Since it inhibits the absorption of fat, the absorption of fat-soluble vitamins can be affected. Weight loss induced by Xenical® is accompanied by improvement in glycemic control. Hence, it is indicated for the obese Type 2 diabetic.

- *Bitter melon extract and Cinnamon extract.* Chinese herbalists have been using bitten melon and cinnamon in treating diabetes for many years with success. Cinnamon extract also has the ability to lower cholesterol. Apparently cinnamon helps to improve diabetic control by increasing the insulin sensitvity[2-3]. Scientists from the USDA were able to identify a molecule in cinnamon that mimics insulin and is responsible for its hypoglycemic properties. Cinnamon has demonstrated both anti-inflammatory and anti-oxidant properties in in vitro cell cultures. In animal studies, cinnamon has been shown to increase HDL cholesterol levels. Bitter melon may stimulate insulin secretion, increase thermogenesis and assist in weight loss. One hundred grams of bitter melon contains 2 grams of fiber and 2 grams of net-carb. It really tastes bitter in cooking and you have to acquire a taste for it. In addition, you have to eat it consistently to have any medicinal effect. It will be easier to take the supplement form. Natural Health Products such as CMX™ contains both cinnamon and bitter melon extracts that can assist patients in controlling diabetes and hypercholesterolemia. Attempts have been made to incorporate CMX™ in our daily food products such as chocolate, yogurt, cereal, beverages and snack bars.

References:

1. Futterweit W. Viewpoint on PCOS, Endocrine News August 2004.

2. Bitter Gourd (Momordica charantia): A dietary approach to hyperglycemia. Nutr Rev July 2006;64:331-7.

3. Khan MS, Alam S, Mahpara A, et al. Cinnamon improves glucose and lipids of people with Type 2 diabetes. Diabetes Care 2003;26:3215-8.

15 : Pros and Cons of Different Diets

There is no single diet that can fit everyone's needs, even with medications. You have to find out for yourself which diet fulfills your needs the most. It also depends on why you became obese in the first place. People gain weight because of overeating, lack of exercise, genetic disorders, stress, or a combination of the above. No single diet can address all the causes at the same time. If a particular diet plan promises you that it can cure all your problems and it sounds too good to be true, it is probably too good to be true. Remember that most of these commercial programs are usually the one program-fits-all type. If you have medical conditions or are on medications, you should consult your doctor first before you attempt these diets on your own. For example, if you are on diuretics and suffering from high blood pressure you should not be eating salt. The sample diets listed in those books will not take that into consideration.

Keep in mind that a diet that helps you to lose weight may not be the right diet to help you to treat your medical conditions.

This chapter lists some of the more commonly followed diets for your reference. It is not the intention to attack those diets but simply to inform the patients of the pros and cons of different diet programs so that they can make better decisions.

Canada's Food Guide Type Diets

Opponents of the quick weight loss diets always say that those diets are unhealthy and it is healthier to go for slow and steady weight loss. The approach is usually associated with eating according to the Food Pyramid or the Food Rainbow, and exercise for 30-60 minutes, seven days a week. In the real world, however, who has time to do this amount of exercise? If people eat according to the food guide but do not do the necessary exercise, they can actually gain weight instead. This approach may be good for healthy people who wish to maintain their weight. For those people who need to lose a lot of fat in order to correct their ailments they will find it to be too slow and easily give up. Eating healthy may not improve diabetic control (see chapter 19). The *DASH (Dietary Approach to Stop Hypertension) diet* is recommended by the American Heart Association and National Institute of Health to combat hypertension and cholesterol. It is similar to the Food Guide except that it recommends less saturated fat and dairy products. Sodium is set at around 2300 mg per day. This diet suggests that when needed, lower the daily sodium intake to 1500 mg per day. It emphasizes fruits, vegetables, fat-free or low-fat milk and milk products. It reduces lean red meat, sweets, added sugar and sweetened drinks. The allowable carbohydrate is set at 55% of daily calorie intake.

Jenny Craig Diet

The *Jenny Craig Diet* is a calorie restrictive diet and follows the principle of Canada's Food Guide. This diet believes that a well balanced diet with fewer calories will lead to weight loss. Sixty percent of the calories will be coming from carbohydrate sources. The diet emphasizes fruits, whole grains, reduced fat dairy products and no sugar added products. In order to lose weight, the client has to eat a low calorie diet. The initial diet plan is about 1000 to 1200 calories per day, and their food products can be expensive. It is convenient for people who have no time to prepare their own meals.

Weight Watcher's Diet

The *Weight Watcher's Diet* plan is an example of a low-calorie low-fat high-fiber diet following the principle of the Canada's Food Guide. Instead of counting portions, the client counts points. Each food item is assigned a certain number of points. There are no banned foods. The client is allowed to eat up to a certain predetermined number of points per day. The number of points allowed usually adds up to less than 1200 calories per day. The theory is that if the client is eating a calorie-restricted diet, no matter which food group the client chooses, as long as the total calorie does not exceed the allowed amount, then the client should be able to lose weight.

Sarah Ferguson, the well-know Duchess of York, is the spokesperson for this diet plan. She said that in order to lose weight, diet itself is not enough. Lifestyle changes (exercise and portion control) are very important to achieve the long-term goal. Since this is calorie restrictive diet with no banned food, the rate of weight loss can be slow. This diet is not disease specific. As you lose weight, you may have to lower your total amount of points in order to be able to lose more weight, or you have to increase the amount of exercise. According to a study done by Heshka S et al, patients who follow the Weight Watcher's diet lost a mean of 4.3 kg at one year and 2.9 kg at two years[3]. The rate of weight loss is slow.

Weight Watchers also has its own line of food products. They are deemed to be unhealthy by some nutritionists because of the amount of additives in them.

All these types of diet are examples of a "healthy diet" that can help people to lose weight. However, it is not supervised by physician, not even dietitian; they may not be suitable for people with complicated medical problems such as diabetes or coronary heart disease. For obese patients who come to see us and have no weight-related medical problems, we usually suggest that they follow a Weight Watchers type of diet. Another good thing about this diet program is that they have frequent group meetings to offer emotional support for each other. Studies have proven that the amount of weight loss is proportional to the number of clinic visits.

South Beach Diet

Dr. Arthur Agatston, a cardiologist, designed this diet to help his cardiac patients to improve on their cholesterol and insulin. The South Beach Diet is a variation of the Atkins diet with the exception of being low fat also. However, Dr. Agatston does not wish to use low-fat-low-carb to describe his diet. The daily intake of carbohydrates in the first phase is about 60-80 grams. It is higher than the Atkins diet. It allows low-fat cheese, non-fat milk (lactose is allowed), creamy Caesar dressing, tomato, beans, artichokes, nuts, water chestnuts, peanut butter and vegetable juice even at the onset of the diet. It tries to avoid saturated fat found in fatty meat but not from cheese. This is not a low-sodium diet. Some recipes in his book contain over 1000 mg of sodium per serving. Caffeine is not encouraged. Apples, sweet potatoes, bran muffins and fat-free pudding are reintroduced in Phase 2. Carrots are to be avoided. The diet allows you to eat white bread or potato immediately after exercise to replenish the glycogen storage. There is no mention about ketosis. Rumor has it that Bill and Hiyeonllary Clinton were on this diet at one time. This is an alternative diet for people who cannot tolerate a strict low-carb diet. However, if you need to eat a low-sodium diet, this is not it.

Mediterranean Diet

Greek people who eat a diet consisting of fish, fruits, nuts, vegetables, legumes, cereals and wine were found to have a lower risk of developing cancer or heart disease. The diet is full of fruits, vegetables and monounsaturated fats. This diet's ability to lower the risk of cancer or heart disease may be due to the lifestyle of the people living in the

Mediterranean area. People's lives in this region are more relaxed and less stressful. Although this diet may be healthy, it may not allow you to lose weight. A diet known as *Low-Fat Lies, High-Fat Frauds and the Healthiest Diet in the World* written by the doctors of Brown University employs the diet of the inhabitants of the Greek Island of Crete. They recommend that people should drink at least two glasses of red wine per day, limit red meat and must exercise daily for 45 minutes. My feeling of this diet is that people can follow it as a healthy lifestyle but should not expect to lose weight fast.

Doctor Supervised Very Low Calorie Diet

This type of diet relies on maintaining a diet is a very low in calories. There is no definition of a "very low calorie" diet. Dr. Luigi Fontane of Washington University in St. Louis call a diet that consumes 1400-2000 calories per day as a very low-calorie diet[1]. Delight Medical Center defines a very low calorie diet (VLCD) as a medical management program where patients consume 800-1100 calories per day[2]. Dr. Leonie Heilbronn of the Pennington Biomedical Research Center, the Louisiana State University defines VLDC as 890 calories per day diet[3]. At the University of California Los Angeles (UCLA), they define their VLCD diet as a diet that consumes 400-1000 calories per day[4]. A very low calorie diet can be defined as a diet that consumes less than 800 calories per day or calorie that is less than 50% of the resting metabolic rate. Some clinics give thier clients B6 and B12 injections three times per week, apparently to help the patient to burn fat. Some patients of the clinic belived that the injection would be given to the area that needs to lose the most. The ability of B vitamin injection as a weight lost aid is not well documented in medical literature. According to the Compendium of Pharmaceuticals and Specialties, "fat burning" is not listed as indications of B12 or B6 vitamin injections. If you can lose weight by simple vitamin injections, why do no other physicians do that for their patients?

Because of the very low calorie intake, it is not unusual to lose 20 pounds per month. According to dietitians, the very low calorie diet is low in all food groups and may not be nutritionally balanced[5-6].

With negative energy balance, weight will be lost. Some clinics claims that only fat weight will be lost on this diet, not muscle weight. No bodily fluid will be lost either. These clinics say that it is achieved by a unique combination of vitamins and supplements. In all the biochemisty and physiology books that I read, when a person eat less than the basal metabolic rate, the body has to go through gluconeogenesis to provide the necessary energy to fuel the body[7-8]. During gluconeogenesis, there is fat burning. However, muscle is also being burned to provide the necessary calorie. This is not a unique phenomenon to the very low calorie diet, but occurs in any weight loss diet, even the high protein diet. During the first one to two weeks of a very low calorie diet, the body will utilize glycogen, amino acids and fatty acids as its energy source. This means that there will be a net loss of muscle in addition to fat loss. Even if you are eating protein from the very beginning, you cannot avoid this muscle loss. If you continue with a very low-calorie type diet without the addition of extra protein, more muscle will be lost. You can regain all the muscle once you have a steady intake of good quality protein in doses of 50-80 g per day[9-10].

If you have two groups of subjects eating two types of very-low-calorie diets with equal amount of calories, one group with high protein and the second group with high carbohydrates, the former group will lose a small amount of muscle and the second group will demonstrate further muscle wasting. For some patients, it may be difficult to maintain this low calorie intake for a prolonged period of time. Once the client goes off the diet, he or she is bound to increase the calorie intake and regain some of the fat weight.

Most very low calorie diet program is under the supervision of nurses and physicians, which is a minimum requirement for a very low calorie diet. Patients should not attempt this type of diet on their own without the proper supervision.

Most diet programs tell their clients to increase the amount of exercise. In some of the low calorie diet clinic, there is no mention on exercise recommendations except patients were told to stay active[6].

As heard on some of the radio ad, "you will lose 20 pounds monthly, month after month". On some web site, it said that you would lose four to five pounds of fatty tissue per week. It did not comment on the type of client that can lose 20 pounds per week. One has to assume it is for an average obese patient with an average height. In order to lose 20 pounds as promised since the diet promises that no muscle or fluid will be lost; the client has to lose 5 pounds of *fat* per week[11]. According to medical literature, patients have to consume 500 calories less than their basal metabolic rate in order to lose 1 pound of fat per week. To lose 5 pounds per week, patient will need to consume 2500 calories less than their basal metabolic rate. The basal metabolic rate of an average build male that is 5 foot 11 inches tall and weights 238 pounds has an estimated metabolic rate of about 2204 calories. In order for him to lose 5 pounds per week, even with complete fasting he has to exercise to burn off another 300 calories per day to reach that goal. In such a diet program, it stated that exercise is not needed. They said that their clients consume at least 850 calories per day without exercising and still lose 20 pounds per week. Even with the lower quote he gives regarding weight loss of 16 pounds of *fat* per month, this patient has to eat 2000 calories less than his basal metabolic rate per day. This equals to a 204 calorie per day diet.

It was reported by registered dietitians that if the patients follows the menu list on the very low calorie diet manual, the daily calorie would be less than 800[5,13,14,15].

Let us look at a female with a height of four foot eleven inches and a weight of 156 pounds (BMI 32.6), her estimated basal metabolic rate is only 1411 calories. Even without eating, she cannot lose 4 pounds of fat per week if she does not do exercise.

There are a few more sample menus but the ones tested all have less than 850 calories per day. The weight lost clinic wishes to define a very low calorie diet as a diet that is lower than 800 calories per day. If their patients are really eating 850 calories or more per day, and that the patients will only lose fat weight, how can the patients lose 5 pounds of fat per week? The calories did not add up.

Meal	Food item	Calories (according to USDA website)
Table 26. Example menus copied from a Very Low Calorie Diet Manual.		
Tuesday Breakfast	¼ cantaloupe 2 Triscuits	48 80
Tuesday Lunch	6 egg whites 8 oz lettuce, celery and cucumber	102 36
Tuesday Dinner	3.5oz veal 8 oz mushrooms, zucchini and tomatoes 2 Triscuits 1 apple 8 oz lettuce, celery and cucumber	108 50 80 73 20 **Total: 597 calories**
Saturday Breakfast	1 orange 1 breadstick	62 40
Saturday Lunch	3.5oz fish 8 oz cabbage	100 55
Saturday Dinner	3.5oz chicken 8 oz green beans and green peppers 1 peach	113 52 42 **Total: 504 calories**

The weight lost clinic said that with the special vitamin B6 and B12 injections, and supplements, the body's metabolism is supposed to improve. By how much can they increase the metabolic rate? There is no formal metabolic study that is known of to back up the claim that B vitamin injections can lead to fat lost in any significant amount. It should be an extremely simple study to do. Even if it is true that the vitamins and supplements can improve on the metabolic rate, how much was the increase? In order to lose 5 pounds of fat per week doing no exercise, and eating a diet that is more than 850 calories per day, the vitamins and supplements have to able to boost the metabolic rate by over 1000 calories per day. Is it possible?

According to medical literature, during a semi-starvation-type diet, the level of triiodothyronine (T3) decreases within a few days and the serum level of an inactive metabolite, reverse T3, rises. This may lead to lower resting energy expenditure.

There are successful stories as shown by the before and after pictures on some of these web sites. However, there are no statistics to show the success rate of patients keeping the weight off.

An "eat-less" diet will always work. However, the key is for you to keep the diet forever. People who lose weight with any diet plan have to keep the weight off as a permanent lifestyle change. Do not give up dieting all together, or you will end up gaining all the weight back, maybe even more.

Dr. Atkins' Diet

This is an example of a low-carbohydrate high-fat high-salt diet. Dr. Atkins proposed that eating carbohydrates is why people gain fat. His diet was found to produce more weight loss than the traditional low-calorie, low-fat diet. However, this diet allows a lot of saturated fat like bacon, whole egg, and cheese, etc. It drew much criticism from the medical community. Patients who went on this diet on their own were able to lose a good amount of weight. The triglycerides level was lowered too. However, the cholesterol, especially the LDL, may come back high. The company is promoting their own line of low-carb products. You should not look at the carbohydrate content only. You also have to be aware of the cholesterol and the saturated fat levels too.

A 60 grams Atkins Advantage™ protein bar contains 9.8 grams of fat. Out of the 9.8 grams of fat, 6.3 grams are *saturated fat*, considered bad fat, worsening your LDL cholesterol level. The company has newer products with lower fat contents.

If your cholesterol is very low, this diet may be suitable for you. Dr. Atkins said that you could eat the excessive amount of fat only if you are *not* eating carbohydrates with it. For people who are not following his diet carefully, eating that amount of fat will worsen the lipid profile. If you follow any diet program, you have to follow it 100%.

The Atkins diet is also high in salt since it allows you to eat salty food such as bacon and cheese.

The Zone Diet

Dr. Barry Sears, the author of the Zone Diet, also identifies carbohydrates as the cause of obesity. He pointed out that the body can only store so much carbohydrates, and excess amounts of carbohydrate will be stored as fat. He does not want his diet to be classified as a low-carbohydrate high-protein diet. In his book, he teaches people what to eat to stay in the "zone". He proposed that the 60% of carbohydrate proportions in the Food Pyramid are too high and he lowered the carbohydrate to 40% of the total calories in his diet plan. At the same time, he increased the amount of protein to 30% with fat staying at 30%. The ratio of the calories from protein to carbohydrate should be 0.75 to get into the "zone". It is very difficult to do the calculation with every meal. This diet does not promote weight loss easily and the diet plan did not make such a claim either. Any weight loss will be due to calorie restrictions. However, we found the approach of the Zone diet quite suitable as a maintenance diet plan.

Protein Power Plan

Designed by Dr. Michael and Mary Dan Eades, husband and wife, the Protein Power Plan is an example of a low-carbohydrate-high-protein diet. They identify insulin as the hormone that causes weight gain. They advise taking potassium supplements, vitamins A, C, E, and B complex, folic acid, iron, magnesium, and calcium. The authors want you do weight training exercises. The idea is that the more muscle you build, the larger quantity of fat you can burn.

They suggest that many autoimmune diseases could be caused by a case of mistaken identity. When the body reacts to the plant proteins of grain products, as these proteins leak through the intestinal wall, the reaction causes harm to our own body structures. Examples of autoimmune diseases are Crohn's disease, ulcerative colitis, rheumatoid arthritis, lupus, psoriasis, Type 1 diabetes, and multiple sclerosis. Placing the patient on a low carbohydrate diet, and eliminating grain products, may help patients with autoimmune diseases to control their symptoms. This diet inspired me to look into the principle of the high protein diet.

The Scarsdale Diet

The late Dr. Tarnower, a cardiologist, was the founder of the Scarsdale Medical Center in New York. This diet is an example of a high-protein low-fat and calorie-restrictive diet. In the beginning of the diet, your intake will be around 1000 calories per day. It is supposed to be a 14 day diet plan. Grapefruit is used daily to help you to burn fat. You are to avoid using oil in cooking. The meal plan is very restrictive also. Allowed food include cold cuts, fruits, lean red meat, egg and low-fat cheese. Banned foods include potatoes, pasta, legumes, corn, peas, regular dairy products, alcohol and all desserts. They do allow veggies and fruits to munch between meals and one alcoholic drink per day. This diet is supposed to bring you into ketosis. There is no maintenance plan per se, but there is a keep trim program that allows more food variety and where wine is allowed.

The Schwarzbein Principle

This is an example of a low-carbohydrate high-fat high-protein diet designed by Dr. Diana Schwarzbein, an endocrinologist, to combat Type 2 diabetes. She believes that the traditional low-fat high-carbohydrate diet causes more weight gain. Banned foods include all processed and refined food, alcohol, salt, caffeine, and artificial sweeteners. She stresses "real" food rather than processed food. Most fat is allowed, such as butter and eggs. A daily exercise routine is suggested. She points out that hyperinsulinemia, caused by eating too much carbohydrates, promotes aging, weight gain, arthritis, diabetes, heart disease, some cancers, and depression. She promotes hormone replacement therapy for post-menopausal women.

References:

1. http://record.wustl.edu/news/page/normal/6447.html

2. www.delightmedical.com/medical-weight-loss-beverly-hills-bakersfield/

3. Heilbronin LK, Jonge LD, Frisard ML, et al. Effect of 6-month calorie restriction on biomarkers of longevity, metabolic adaptation, and oxidative stress in overweight individuals. A randomized controlled trial. JAMA 2006;295:1539-48.

4. http://rfoweightloss.med.ucla.edu/body.cfm?id=32&oTopID=31

5. www.Nutrimundo.com/diets/dr_bernstein_diet.html

6. www.thedietlibrary.com/DrBernsteinDiet.html?b=5596

7. Salway JG, Metabolism at a Glance, Third edition, Blackwell Publishing. 2004:54.

8. Harrison's Principles of Internal Medicine, 10th edition, page 493-495.

9. Gelfand RA, Hendler R. Diabetes Metab Rev 1989; 5:17-30.

10. Vazqueq JA, Kazi U, Madani N. Am J Clin Nutr 1995;62:93-103.

11. Heshka S, Anderson JW, Atkinson RL, et al. Weight loss with self-help compared with a structured commercial program: A randomized trial. JAMA 2003;289(14):1792-8.

12. www.drbdiet.ca/as/DrBProfile

13. www.cbc.ca/consumers/market/files/health/Bernstein_diet/

14. www.steadyhealth.com/dr_bernstein_s_health_and_diet_clinic_toronto_t55560.html

15. Sarah Scott. Chatelaine April 2004;64-74.

"Yo-yo dieting is worse than no dieting"

16: VITAL STATISTICS

Date of first visit:

Weight: _____kg (_____pounds)

Height: _____cm (_____inches)

Neck Size: _____ cm (_____inches)

Blood Pressure: _____

Body Mass Index: _____

Percentage of Body Fat: _____%

Total Amount of Body Fat: _____ pounds

Blood Sugar: _____

Hemoglobin A1c: _____

Triglycerides: _____

Total Cholesterol: _____ HDL:_____ LDL:_____ Ratio: _____

ALT (SGOT): _____

After two months of dieting:

Weight: _____kg (_____pounds)

Height: _____cm (_____inches)

Neck Size: _____ cm (_____inches)

Blood Pressure: _____

Body Mass Index: _____

Percentage of Body Fat: _____%

Total Amount of Body Fat: _____ pounds

Blood Sugar: _____

Hemoglobin A1c: _____

Triglycerides: _____

Total Cholesterol: _____ HDL:_____ LDL:_____ Ratio: _____

ALT (SGOT): _____

17: PHASE ONE INDUCTION PHASE

This diet can be classified as a low-sodium low-carbohydrate low-fat high-protein high-fiber diet. There are three phases to this diet:

PHASE 1. INDUCTION PHASE

PHASE 2. CONTINUED WEIGHT LOSS PHASE

PHASE 3. MAINTENANCE PHASE

The amount of time you need to stay on with each phase of the diet varies. It varies with your commitment, your body's response, and your goal. The amount of fat and sodium allowed in all three phases remains relatively constant. The objective of the first phase of the diet is to use up the glycogen stored in the muscle and liver. Your metabolism will be changed from fat forming into fat burning. Once we are sure that you are using fat as the main source of energy, you can move into Phase 2. During Phase 2, you will try to find out how much carbohydrates you can tolerate while still burn fat. You will be given additional amounts of carbohydrate to eat and your rate of fat loss will be monitored. More and more carbohydrate will then be added to your diet as long as you show a good amount of fat loss. The objective is to lose 1 to 2 pounds of fat weekly or have a 10% of weight loss in 8 weeks. Exercise is encouraged. Different people can tolerate different amounts of carbohydrate in their diet. Gender, age, muscle mass, activity, mood, stress, exercise, and medications are some of the factors that can affect the metabolism. Phase 3 will allow you to eat carbohydrates in much higher quantities without regaining the weight.

Phase 1. Induction Phase

This is the beginning of your diet and it is the most important phase of the diet. It requires total compliance on your part or it will fail. You will be starting with a very low carbohydrate count, usually no more than *20 grams* per day. You do not have to count the actual amount of carbohydrates in the foods that you are going to eat. Just follow the diet plan and you will be within the limit. Since you know now that your daily carbohydrate allowance is only 20 grams, when you read the food labels (Chapter 12) while shopping at the supermarket, you can decide if that item is good for your diet or not. After two weeks on this diet, your body chemistry will be manipulated by the food that you consumed to burn fat rather than store it. The fat burning will occur 24 hours a day around the clock, even while you are sleeping. This is why this diet allows you to lose weight and inches quickly. When glycogen is metabolized, it releases the trapped water and patients may experience an increase in urinary frequency. You will end up with 7 to 10 pounds of weight loss (fat and water) in the first two weeks. We utilize a body analyzer in our offices to assess the patient's fat and water weight so that we can tell if the patient is losing fat, water or both. However, you may not have this kind of equipment at home. You can tell that you lost water because if your shoes fit looser and your ring is not as tight as before. You can tell that you lost fat when your clothing fits differently A small amount of muscle will also be metabolized, make sure that you eat your proteins.

First Appointment

Before we enroll you in the diet program, we have to do a medical history and any physical examination as needed on you to make sure that this is the right program for you.

- You need to tell us your past medical and weight history

- You need to tell us your current list of medications

- You need to have your blood pressure checked

- You need to have your blood tested so that we have a baseline value for your kidney function, glucose, hemoglobin, liver, thyroid, cholesterol, triglycerides, uric acid, ferritin and serum electrolytes. If you are diabetic, you might need to be checked for yeast in the vagina, insulin levels, microalbumin, A1c and C-peptide. If you have signs of Cushing's Syndrome, you will need a 24-hour urine test, ACTH level, and serum cortisone test. If you have significant heart disease, you will need an ECG (check QT interval), echocardiogram (check cardiomyopathy, left and right ventricular hypertrophy), and a highly sensitive C-Reactive Protein test (hsCRP). If you have polycystic ovary syndrome, you will need fasting insulin, FSH, LH, testosterone, DHEA and pelvic ultrasound. Sometime we can obtain these results from your family doctor or specialist prior to your appointment

- You *cannot* go on this diet if you have significant kidney disease (GFR<40), significant liver disease or Type 1 diabetes on insulin. If you are pregnant or breast feeding, do not go on this diet without the doctor's supervision. Patients with celiac disease may not be good candidates either since some of the diet bread for Phase two is high in gluten. Patients who are Type 2 diabetics taking insulin will be assessed by the physician first before they go on the diet. A blood test called C-peptide will be ordered to check if the patient produces enough insulin. In my experience, 87% of the obese Type 2 diabetics on insulin produce adequate amounts of insulin themselves[1]. Vegans have to modify the Phase 1 diet to satisfy their dietary restrictions. They have to accept the fact that they will not lose weight as quickly as other patients

- Your height and weight will be measured and your *Body Mass Index* (BMI) and percent body fat calculated. Normally, only patients with BMI of higher than 30 (27 for Asians and East Asians) before they are accepted into our program. In addition to your weight, you need to have at least one medical condition that is associated with obesity before you are accepted into the program. If there is a strong family history (first-degree relatives) of Type 2 diabetes, premature coronary heart disease or cardiovascular events (having the disease before the age of 55 is considered as premature), you will also qualify for the program. You will be accepted if you have a surgical procedure planned for the near future and the surgeon requires you to lose some weight before going to the operating room

- Your n*eck circumference and/or waist circumference* will be measured. We use an Impedance Scale to measure the percentage of body fat

(Weight in kg) x (% of body fat) = total body fat in kg

- You will receive counseling for the Phase 1 portion of the diet (Fat Burning Induction Phase) if you qualify. We expect you to follow the diet 100% and not to deviate from the diet plan. The supervising physician has the right to discharge the patient from the program if the patient is not following the rules of the diet program

- You will be given a urine sample bottle to take home. Collect a *fasting* sample (the first urine sample in the morning before eating or drinking) and bring it back to us on the day of your return visit, usually two weeks. You do not have to refrigerate the sample

We have tried to make this diet plan simple. You do not have to count calories and most of the time you do not have to count carbohydrates. Just follow the instructions and you will be eating within the limit. You do not have to buy expensive food. A shopping list is provided in this manual so that you can do one-stop shopping. Learn to read food labels correctly. The nutrition values on the label tell you the amount of carbohydrate *per serving*, and not for the whole contents. Do not be fooled. If you cannot find the right type of food item as listed, do not buy them since it will either be higher in carbohydrate or salt. Look into specialty stores or on the internet such as www.ontarionutrition.ca for those food items.

Objectives of the Phase 1 Diet:

- To use up all the stored glucose (glycogen) in the body, which usually takes about 2 to 3 days, faster if you exercise

- To eliminate some of the excess body water

- To utilize fat as the major source of energy (lipolysis)

- To minimize lean muscle loss

- To consume as little carbohydrate as possible (less than 1-2 g of net-carbohydrates per serving, and not more than a total of 20 g per day)

- To consume as little saturated and trans-fats as possible

- To consume less than 1500 mg of sodium per day and less than 170 mg of sodium per serving

- To lose 7 to 10 pounds by following a diet that is low in sugar, starch, bad fat and sodium

- To achieve these goals within 2 weeks

There are three lists in Phase 1. List 1 shows what you can *eat as much as and as often as you want.* List 2 shows you the food items that you are allowed in small quantities only. List 3 shows you food items that you should avoid while on Phase 1.

List #1. Foods that you can eat as much as you desire and you can eat them at anytime of the day:

- Any type of meat, including red, dark and white meats. They have to be *extra-lean* when you consume them. When possible, remove the fat and skin before or after cooking. Ground meats from beef, chicken or turkey have to be the extra-lean variety (<10% fat). Regular ground beef is 30% fat and lean ground beef is 17% fat

- *Low-sodium* fat-free chicken or turkey breast deli meat. They can be difficult to find. They are not pre-packaged and you have to ask the worker at the deli counter if the supermarket is carrying this kind of product. Do not just go for fat-free deli meats because they are usually very high in sodium

- Any kind of fish, including the fatty type since it contains essential fatty acids. Fish has to be either fresh or frozen without added salt

- Scallops. They have very little fat and cholesterol

- Egg whites. They are pure protein without salt, fat, cholesterol and carbohydrate. It has the best amount of quality protein out of all protein sources

- Green leafy vegetables. As long as it is green in color and is the leafy part, you can have it. There are too many to list individually. Go to the supermarket and find it yourself. Cabbage is allowed but not brussel sprouts because it is higher in carbohydrates

- Olive oil and canola oil. These oils have high amounts of monounsaturated fatty acids (60%) and better omega-3 to omega-6 ratios (2 to 1) when compared to other vegetable oils

- Any kind of sweetener. Splenda® is preferred because you can cook or bake with it. You can also use stevia, a natural sweetener that has recently been approved by the FDA to use in food products. Xylitol and Erythitol are sugar alcohols that can be used as sweetners.

- Diet drinks, including pop, Crystal Light®, diet iced tea, coffee, black tea, herbal tea and green tea. Try to choose the type with low sodium and low caffeine contents

- Jell-O Light® jelly or similar products (not the Jell-O pudding)

- Calorie-free fruit spread but not "No sugar added" jam

- Shirataki® noodles or Tofu Shirataki® noodles. They are mainly fiber and contain minimal amounts of sugar and starch

- Low-sodium vegetable broth or bouillon, low-sodium chicken or beef broth

- Spices and herbs, as long as they do not contain salt. For example, Mrs. Dash®, McCormick® Spices, black pepper, white pepper, paprika and curry powder etc

- Xanthan gum or guar gum (to make gravy and to thicken soup, see our cookbook for more detail)

List #2: Here is a list of food items that you can eat in *limited quantities* everyday. However, you need to be careful with the quantity:

- Shellfish. Such as 1 small lobster tail or 5 large headless shrimps

- BranCrispbread® from Norway is high in fiber and low in starch. Two pieces three times per day

- Very low-carb Flexseed Bread with 1 gram of net-carb. One slice twice a day. Available at speciality store like OntarioNutrition.ca

- Egg yolk. 1 per day (watch your intake if you have elevated serum cholesterol)

- Calorie-free dressings, such as BBQ sauce, ketchup (1 tsp per serving)

- Table cream 5-10% or soy creamer. 5 ml (1 tsp) per regular cup of coffee or tea

- Low-carb cookie or biscotti, one piece every 4 hours

- Sugar-free gum, candy, gummy bears, halva, marshmallow, meringues and chocolate. Limit to 5 to 10 g of sugar alcohols per serving. You can have 1 serving every 4-5 hours. Try to pick the kind that is also fat-free. Too much sugar alcohol can cause diarrhea. The response is different for different people. Pick only 1 snack at a time and not to exceed 4 snacks per day.

- Other fresh vegetables. A total of not more than four cups of alfalfa, artichoke hearts, asparagus, cauliflower, celery, cucumber, mushrooms, green bell peppers, green onion, broccoli, green (string) beans, wax beans, zucchini, bean sprouts, and eggplant per day. You do not have to measure them physically. We want you to know that these vegetables have higher carbohydrate contents than green leafy vegetables; hence, it is not all you can eat. Please note that the following are not allowed: corn, peas, tomatoes, leek and legumes (lentil beans, pinto beans, lama beans, navy beans etc)

- Ginger, lemon, lime and garlic for cooking

- Low-sodium soy sauce, teriyaki sauce and Half Salt® to taste

- Canned fish. Must be labeled as "Low-sodium in water" tuna or salmon and not more than a total of two cans per week because of the risk of mercury contamination. Avoid "tuna in water"

- Sugar-free popsicle. One per serving

- Protein shakes. The best type of protein shake comes from egg protein. Do not use it more than once a day

- SMAPS® cereal. Half a cup of this cereal contains 2 net-carbohydrates. Since dairy products are not allowed on Phase 1, you have to eat it dry, like a snack, or take it with cold coffee and cream, or take it with half a cup of egg protein shake

List #3: Foods that you should avoid (do not use) on Phase 1:

- Foods with high salt content. Most canned foods, most deli meats, processed meat, smoked meat or smoked fish, non-diet sauces, and pickled foods (Table 27). These restrictions are particularly important for people who are suffering from high blood pressure, diabetes, water retention, congestive heart failure, and declined kidney function

- Any vegetables that are grown underneath the ground (root vegetables), but you may use garlic and ginger in your cooking

- Most dairy and non-dairy products, except a small amount of cream is allowed for coffee and tea. One cup of milk has 12 g of sugar (lactose) and one serving of cream has only 1 g of sugar

- Breaded foods or deep fried foods

- Sugar. Including glucose, fructose, sucrose, galactose, maltose

- Flour products such as bread, pasta, ordinary noodles

- Starches such as potatoes, yam, rice, dry beans (legumes) and their products

- Fruits. One banana has an amount of sucrose equivalent to 8 teaspoons of sugar. You may use some lemon and lime for cooking and drinking

- Juice of all kinds. One cup of freshly squeezed orange juice has 4 teaspoons of sugar

- Alcohol of all kinds. Alcohol is not a carbohydrate but it carries 7 empty calories per gram. Beer has high amounts of carbohydrate and is not suitable for this diet

- Any food that is allowed in Phase 2 and 3 will not be allowed in Phase 1. Please read Phase 2 and Phase 3 shopping lists in the subsequent chapters

These restrictions are for Phase 1. We will re-introduce some other food items into your diet once you are in Phase 2 and 3.

There is no set breakfast menu, lunch menu or dinner menu. Eat only the right kinds of food and do not over eat. There is no need to count calories. You should include some protein every time you eat. That is, do not eat only vegetables and no protein. If you are unsure of a certain food item that you could not locate in this chapter, the answer will be -

Table 27. Food that has Low Carbohydrate Content, Glycemic Load, and Calories that is Suitable for the Induction Phase (Fat Off)

Alfalfa sprout	Lettuce
Asparagus	Lamb chops
Bacon, peameal*	Lemon (in cooking)
Bean sprouts	Lobster tail
Beef broth*	Low cal dressing
Beef jerky*	Mushroom
Beef pastrami*	Mustard
Bok choy	Oil, olive or canola
Broccoli	Pepper, green
Cabbage	Perch
Calamari	Pickles*
Cauliflower	Pork chops
Celery	Pork tenderloin
Chicken	Radish
Chicken Broth*	Ribs (with low-carb BBQ sauce)
Club soda	Roast beef
Cod	Sardines (fresh)
Coffee	Sashimi
Crab meat (not the imitation kind)	Scallops
Crystal light®	Shrimp meat
Cucumber	Soy sauce (low sodium)
Curry paste (low sodium)	Sole
Diet soda	Spinach
Duck breast	Squid
Egg, white	Steak
Eggplant	Salmon (fresh or low-sodium)
Game hen	Salmon, canned or smoked*
Garlic (in cooking)	Sugar free candy
Green beans	Tea
Green bell peppers	Tuna, light in water*
Green onion	Turkey
Ham*, lean	Turkey breast, deli*
Half and half cream	Vinegar
Hamburger, extra lean	Veal
Herbs and spices	Watercress
Hot pepper	Wax beans
Horse radish	Zucchini

*Avoid if you have high blood pressure or water retention.

do not eat it. One hundred percent compliance is needed to be successful. This is a radical change in your eating habit, if you cannot eat as directed, do not attempt this diet. Yo-yo dieting is worse than no dieting.

Follow These Rules When You Are On This Diet

- *Do not skip meals.* This diet works better if you eat small meals every 3 to 4 hours as compared to complete fasting. The prevalence of obesity is decreased by the number of daily meals[2]. Note that fasting not only increases your fat burning but also increases *protein burning* (bad effect) leading to wasting of lean muscle mass. When you fast, your body will feel stressed and increase your adrenaline secretion. Adrenaline causes an increase in blood glucose by *glycogenolysis* (breaking down of glycogen to form glucose) and *gluconeogenesis* (breakdown of muscle and fat to form glucose). This is why diabetics find their blood glucose goes up and is difficult to control during stressful times. The objective of this diet is to lose fat and not muscle. It is the amount of muscle in your body that controls your body's basal metabolic rate. The larger your muscle mass, the easier for you to lose weight. This is why men can lose weight faster than women. For the same amount of walking, the person with the bigger lean body mass will burn more calories than can someone with less muscle. This is why a person on the calorie-reduction type diet, after losing 10 pounds on a certain number of calories, cannot continue to lose weight. He is losing muscle on this type of diet and his basal metabolism decreases with his weight loss. In order to lose more weight, he has to continue eating less as he loses weight.

Eat a small amount of protein even if you are not hungry in the morning, such as the egg white of a hard-boiled egg or a protein shake. This prevents muscle loss. One of the side effects of a low-protein low-calorie diet is hair loss. Make sure you do not skimp on protein. If there are occasions that you are not able to eat frequent small meals, do not worry. The diet should be able to fit into your lifestyle also. You are not going to quit your job because you have to do this diet.

If you skip meals, you tend to eat a lot at supper. This might cause weight gain even if the total calories you ingested the whole day are the same. For example, if you eat three meals a day and each meal has 500 calories and a glycemic load of 10 (which is considered to be low). This does not affect your blood glucose or insulin. But if you eat only one meal with 1500 calories and a glycemic load of 30 (which is high), this will cause a big rise in blood glucose and trigger an insulin surge.

- *Eat slowly and eat the right type of food only*. Although you may not feel full immediately, you will feel full after 1 to 2 hours. This is because the types of food that you are allowed to eat are digested slowly and the blood glucose does not go up sharply (as compared to a high-carbohydrate, high-glycemic index meal). The main idea of this part of the diet is to minimize the secretion of insulin. If the blood glucose goes up too much or too quickly after you eat, it will trigger the body to secrete more insulin and store calories as fat. Both meat and fat have low glycemic indexes and low glycemic loads.

- *You are allowed to eat three types of protein*. They are *EGG WHITES*, any kind of *LEAN UNPROCESSED MEAT* as long you can separate out the fat from the protein before you eat them (avoid side bacon, hot dogs, fatty ground beef, sausages, or organ meats such as kidney and liver), and *SEAFOOD* (except imitation seafood, mussels, oysters, clams). No legumes, no peanuts, no peanut butter, and no nuts are allowed on Phase 1. It is very important not to have any breaded coating on your food. If you have high cholesterol levels, use the Break Free™ liquid egg product, Egg Creations™ or Omega-Pro™ liquid egg product, or egg whites instead of whole eggs. Meats, such as hot dogs, bacon, ham, regular ground beef and sausages, usually have a lot of fillers or fat or salt and so they are considered to be poor quality meats. They are not recommended. Check the ingredients to make sure they are made of 100% meat. Even if it says 100% meat, read the nutritional information and make sure that there is not too much fat. For example, 100% beef *does not* mean 100% beef protein. Even if 20% of the product is beef fat, it can still be labeled as 100% beef.

We want you to include protein in every meal. Your body needs protein continuously to repair and maintain bodily functions. The ingestion of protein triggers the secretion of glucagon, which counteracts the effects of insulin. We do not allow commercially prepared protein bars that usually have a lot of saturated fat, calories, and chemicals. Although nuts and peanut butter have some protein, they are also full of fat and carbohydrates. Hence, we do not consider them as good sources of protein. An occasional glass of a protein shake that is low in carbohydrates and fat is allowed. However, it is not a substitution for a good protein meal.

Pork chops are not lean when you purchase them from the butcher shop. You may even cook the pork chops with the fat attached. However, you have to trim off all the visible fat before you put it into your mouth. People hesitate to eat meat because they worry about cholesterol. They need to understand that it is the fat attached to the meat that increases your serum cholesterol. Eating the small amount of cholesterol in meat will not increase the serum cholesterol. Remember that it is not the dietary cholesterol that raises the blood LDL cholesterol. High LDL cholesterol level is related to eating saturated and trans fat, sugar and starch. Lean meat is mostly protein.

People were told not to eat lobster, scallops or shrimp because they are high in fat and cholesterol. This is only partially true. The parts of the lobster and shrimp that contain the high amount of fat and cholesterol are located in the head and body. The tails (meat) of the lobster and shrimp contain mainly protein. According to the USDA *Nutrient Database for Standard Reference*, gram for gram, the meat from lobster, scallops or shrimp have less saturated fat than the white meat of chicken or turkey (Table 28). Shrimp meat has higher level of cholesterol than lobster meat but much less saturated fat than beef. The suggested maximum daily cholesterol allowance is 300 mg per day. Unlike essential protein and essential fatty acid, there is no such thing as essential cholesterol. Hence, you do not need to consume any cholesterol at all. Your liver can synthesize cholesterol from sugar or fat. Remember that LDL cholesterol increase from eating too much saturated fat rather than eating cholesterol. If you have to chose, you should choose shellfish over red meat.

Table 28. Cholesterol and Saturated Fat of Meat and Seafood.

Serving Size 3.5 oz	Cholesterol (mg)	Saturated Fat (g)
Egg, 1 whole	212	1.6
Pork loin	85	3.6
Beef, top round	90	2.0
Chicken, light meat	85	1.3
Turkey, light meat	68	1.2
Oysters, 6 whole	38	0.6
Shrimp meat	195	0.3
Lobster meat	72	0.1
Scallop	36	0.1
Crab meat	72	0.1

Table 29 demonstrates to you the fat content of some of the food that you eat. Try to choose the food with the lowest fat content. For example, if you want to eat steak, eat the sirloin cut rather than rib steak. Note that this table gives you the total fat content and does not specify if it is good fat versus bad fat.

Table 29. Fat Content of Commonly Consumed Foods.

Food	Total Fat (g)
Avocados, 1	30
Back bacon, 47 g	4
Breakfast bacon, 32 g	16
Beef, eye-of-round roast, 88 g	6
Beef, flank steak, 86 g	9
Beef, lean ground, 70 g	10
Beef, regular ground, 76 g	16
Beef, rib-eye, 86 g	7
Beef, short ribs, 88 g	31
Beef, tenderloin, 86 g	8
Beef, top sirloin, 86 g	6
Bologna, 42 g	9
Brownies, 36 g	10
Butter, 15 ml	12
Cheesecake, 1 slice	18
Cheeseburgers, 102 g	15
Cheese, Blue, 53 g	15
Cheese, Camembert, 48 g	12
Cheese, cheddar, 52 g	17
Cheese, cheddar light, 42 g	7
Cheese, cream, fat-free, 100 g	1.4
Cheese, feta, 125 ml	17
Cheese, goat, 21% MF, 50 ml	11
Cheese, mozzarella, 125 ml	10
Cheese, parmesan, 125 ml	16
Chicken, no skin, ¼	4
Clams, canned, 125 ml	2
Coconut, shredded, 125 ml	17
Cod, 90 g	1
Crab meat, 125 ml	1
Half and half, 15 ml	2
Croissants, 57 g	12
Danish pastry, 1	13
Doughnuts, 1	16
Duck, no skin, ¼	12
Eggs, 1	5
Fish sticks, 83 g	10
Ham, roasted, 70 g	6
Hamburgers, plain, 90 g	12
Halibut, 159 g	5
Hot dog, beef, 1	9

Food	Total Fat (g)
Hot dog, chicken, 1	7
Kielbasa, 61 g	9
Lamb chops, 92 g	27
Lamb, leg, 88 g	6
Liver, beef, 85 g	7
Liver, chicken, 125 ml	4
Lobster tail, boiled, 125 ml	1
Macaroni and cheese, 250 ml	18
Milk, chocolate, 2%, 250 ml	5
Milk, 1%, 250 ml	3
Milk, 2%, 250 ml	5
Milk, skim, 250 ml	1
Milk, whole, 250 ml	9
Muffins, bran, 50 g	5
Mussels, steamed, 15	2
Nuts, almonds, 125 ml	38
Nuts, cashews, 125 ml	34
Nuts, pine, 125 ml	43
Nuts, pistachios, 125 ml	38
Nuts, walnuts, 125 ml	33
Oils, olive, 15 ml	14
Oysters, steamed, 5	3
Pastrami, 57 g	4
Peanut butter, 30 ml	17
Peanut, roasted, 125 ml	39
Perch, 100 g	2
Pork, back ribs, 70 g	21
Pork, chops, 69 g	7
Pork, loin, 88g	10
Pork, spareribs, 75 g	16
Potato chips, 10	7
Red snapper, 170 g	3
Scallops, 3 large	2
Sunflower seed, 75 ml	20
Shrimp, 10 large	1
Sole, baked, 127 g	2
Soup, chicken noodle, 250 ml	4
Soup, clam chowder, 250 ml	5
Soup, cream of mushroom	13
Soup, split pea, 250 ml	5
Sour cream, 15 ml	2
Soy milk, 250 ml	3
Tofu, soft, 100 g	3
Yogurt, plain, low-fat, 175 g	1

To rank protein sources according to their biological values, we have to find out the highest ratio of essential amino acids as compared to the total amount of protein, gram per gram. The Protein Digestibility Corrected Amino Acid Score (PDCAAS) is a method of evaluating the quality of the amino acid content of a certain protein. There are 11 essential amino acids in human nutrition. Protein sources that have all of the essential amino acids have a PDCAAS score of 1. Poor quality protein has a lower score. The best protein source is albumin (from egg), followed by milk proteins, animal products, legumes, cereals and roots in descending order (Table 30).

Table 30. PDCAAS Score of Some Common Proteins.	
Egg white	1.12
Cheese	1.00
Pork	0.98
Beef	0.97
Whey (protein from milk)	0.96
Casein	0.95
Milk	0.95
Chicken	0.93
Soy	0.91
Pinto bean	0.73
Kidney beans	0.68
Rye	0.68
Whole wheat	0.54
Lentils	0.52
Peanuts	0.52
Gelatin (lack tryptophan)	0.00

Table 31. Compare Nutritional Values when Half-and-Half verse Homo Milk is used to Lighten a Cup of Coffee.					
	Quantity	Calories	Carbo-hydrate	Fat	Protein
Half-and-half 10%MF	1 teaspoon	20	1 g	2 g	0.4 g
Homo milk	4 teaspoon	37	3 g	1.9 g	2 g

- *Use table cream or half-and-half instead of milk to lighten your coffee or tea.* In this part of the diet, we want you to eliminate as much carbohydrate as possible. Dairy products contain milk sugar called *lactose.* In order to achieve the same amount of "whiteness" obtained by one teaspoon of half-and-half cream, you would have to use four times the volume of homo milk.

The net effect is that you will be consuming more carbohydrates and calories when you use milk instead of 10% cream. The amount of fat for both cups of coffee will be similar. Splenda® is your sweetener of choice because it has not been associated with any types of cancer. Since even the half-and-half cream contains 1 g of carbohydrate, limit your coffee intake to 2-3 cups per day. Boiled, unfiltered coffee raises total and LDL cholesterol because coffee beans contain a terpenoid lipid called cafestol. The amount of cafestol in the cup depends on the brewing method. There is no cafestol in paper-filtered drip coffee, but levels are high in the unfiltered coffee that is still widely consumed in Greece, the Middle East and Turkey.

- Eat vegetables that are visible above the ground except tomatoes, corn, peas and legumes (dry beans), etc. Any vegetable that grows underneath the ground should be avoided during Phase 1. Since they are the storage organs for the plant, they store food in the form of starch. Even though two different kinds of vegetables might have similar total carbohydrate counts per standard weight, the effect of these vegetables on the blood glucose level may vary. It is because there are two different types of carbohydrate (absorbable and non-absorbable) in vegetables (Figure 13).

The *absorbable* type of carbohydrate, as found in potatoes, raises blood glucose quickly after ingestion and the body will store any excess carbohydrate as fat. Sugar alcohol is a type of absorbable carbohydrate that gets absorbed slowly; hence, it will not produce an excess rise in blood glucose. However, since sugar alcohol does have calories that you can absorb, it can cause weight gain or make it difficult to loss weight (see Chapter 20, table 44).

The *non-absorbable type*, as found in celery, presents as *fiber* (insoluble) and in apples, presents as *pectin* (soluble). Humans cannot absorb these kinds of carbohydrates and they will be excreted from the bowel undigested. Even though celery has 4 g of carbohydrates listed per stalk, the actual amount of carbohydrate that gets absorbed is low. There is a total of 3 g of fiber and the net-carb is only 1 g. Hence, it has very little effect on raising the blood glucose level after ingestion.

We will be teaching you how to choose the right type of vegetable. We do not mean to say that food like apples, potatoes or corn is bad for your health. However, if you are overweight, it will be more difficult to lose weight when your diet is full of fruits and vegetables that contain highly absorbable carbohydrates and high glycemic loads. Read chapter 12 and chapter 20 to learn to identify the different kinds of nonabsorbable carbohydrates. As a rule of thumb, eat a maximum of four cups of cooked vegetables per day. Do not over eat the cooked vegetables.

Some people consider lentil beans, kidney beans and navy beans as protein. Since this diet allows people to eat as much protein they as desired, they end up eating a lot of legumes on Phase 1. This diet does not allow legumes on Phase 1 because those beans are not high in protein. They are high in carbohydrates with *some* protein in it. Here is a break down of the macro-nutrients of red kidney beans. One quarter cup of boiled red kidney beans consists of 4 g of protein, 10 g of carbohydrate, 3.5 g of fiber, 6.5 g of starch and 0 g of fat. Hence, it has a net-carb of 6.5 g, which is similar to 1.6 teaspoons of sugar. There is more starch than protein. Table 32 compares the net-carb contents of different kinds of beans in relationship to lettuce.

Table 32. Net-carb of Boiled Beans in Relationship to Lettuce[6].					
	Serving Size	Total Carb (g)	Fiber (g)	Net-carb (g)		Equivalent in sugar (tsp)
				Sugar	Starch	
Lettuce	¼ head	4	1.6	2.4	0	0.6
Lentil Bean	½ cup	20	8.0	1.8	10.2	3.0
Barley	½ cup	22	3.0	0.2	18.8	4.8
Kidney Bean	½ cup	20	6.6	0.2	13.2	3.4
Navy Bean	½ cup	24	9.6	0.2	14.2	3.6
Pinto Bean	½ cup	22	7.4	0.2	14.4	3.7
Soybean	½ cup	9	5.0	2.6	1.4	1.0

This table demonstrated that a quarter head of lettuce has an equivalent amount of 0.6 teaspoon of sugar; whereas half a cup of lentil beans has an equivalent amount of 3 teaspoons of sugar. Soybean has the least amount of net-carb among all the legumes and is suitable for Phase 2 consumption.

- *Fight your carbohydrate cravings.* Carbohydrate addiction is a true entity, just like smoking and alcoholism. Females tend to crave carbohydrates more than males. Males crave salty food instead. Craving for carbohydrates is worse before menstrual periods and during the winter time. Seasonal affective disorder suffers gain weight by an increase in carbohydrate cravings. If it is due to hormonal changes, the craving will be self limiting. Sixty eight percent of men and 97% of women report cravings. The higher the BMI, the higher the amount of cravings.

Craving for carbohydrate occur from low blood glucose. If you tough it out and try not to consume any carbohydrates, the blood glucose will be returned to normal through gluconeogenesis (fat and muscle burning). This will take a few days of Phase 1 to accomplish. Once you are burning fat and go into ketosis, the cravings will disappear. Patients need to go through a "carbohydrate withdrawal" period before going into ketosis and before cravings disappear. However, if the patient cheats on carbohydrates, the patient will have to go through the same withdrawal symptoms again. The more you eat, the more you will crave. Not everyone has to go through withdraw, just like quitting cigarette smoking.

- *Drink enough fluids so that your urine appears pale yellow.* Just look at the color of the urine every time you void. If the urine color is very pale yellow, you can stop drinking. Do not over drink. Return to the clinic with a urine sample collected first thing in the morning on the day of your visit, usually two weeks from the beginning of your diet.

- *There is no set menu.* If you can order an "all day breakfast" in a restaurant, what is wrong with an "all day dinner"? If you visit Hong Kong from Canada by plane, there is a time zone different of twelve hours. When you reach Hong Kong at 8 AM local time, which is 8 PM Toronto time, should you eat breakfast or supper? It is breakfast time in Hong Kong but your biological clock is supposed to be super time. To me, it makes no difference, food is food. There is no need to count calories in our diet program. Eat when you are hungry and stop eating when you are full. The numbers on the nutritional food labels determine the suitability of that food item.

Figure 14. Different Types of Carbohydrate.

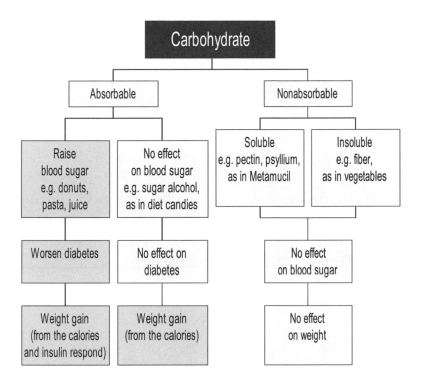

- *Juicing of vegetables and fruits is not good for this diet.* It removes the fiber that helps with regularity and concentrates the absorbable carbohydrates (high glycemic index). For people with constipation or high cholesterol problems, take one or two packages of sugar-free Metamucil, flaxseed, or bran fiber daily. To find out how to calculate the amount of absorbable carbohydrates in the food that you purchased from the supermarket, read Chapter 12. Your vegetables are your main source of carbohydrates. Do not over eat. You are only allowed 20 g of absorbable carbohydrates per day. You need to spread your carbohydrate intake throughout the day. Do not eat all of it in the same meal. Again, this is to minimize the possibility of triggering insulin hyper-secretion.

- *This is a protein and vegetable diet.* Please note that we want you to have some good quality protein every time you eat. This is not a vegetarian diet. Remember that most of your carbohydrates in this part of the diet come from vegetables. Meat, seafood and oils have minimal amounts of carbohydrate only. By adding meat and oil to your vegetables, you can slow down the absorption of the carbohydrate (i.e. to lower the glycemic index - see Chapter 11). *Cholecystokinin* is a hormone that is found in abundance in the cells of the small intestine. When you eat a meal that contains some fat and protein, cholecystokinin is released into the blood stream as the food reaches the small intestine. Cholecystokinin in turn signals the brain to feel full and stop eating. A meal that contains only carbohydrates does not trigger this response. This is one of the reasons why you should have good fat or protein included in your meal every time you eat vegetables.

Figure 15. Fat Metabolism when Ingested With or Without Carbohydrate.

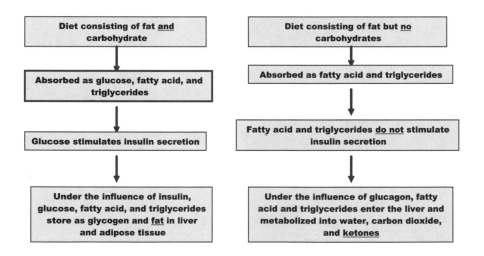

Dr. A Astrup, Dr. W.H. Saris, and Dr. F.M. Sacks presented papers at the Second International Congress on "Prediabetes" and the Metabolic Syndrome in Barcelona, Spain, April 2007. They found that increased protein consumption as compared to carbohydrate increases the satiating power and thermogenic effect of the diet. Keeping the total calories and fat calorie constant, increase protein intake from 12% to 25% of calories produces more weight loss (9.4 kg vs. 5.9Kg) over six months. They pointed out that the DASH diet is too high in carbohydrates (58%), which lowers the HDL levels and does not reduce triglycerides. The OmniHeart study found that a lower carbohydrate version of the DASH diet that emphasized protein or unsaturated fat further reduced blood pressure and LDL cholesterol, and lower triglycerides. Estimated risk reduction was 20% with the carbohydrate rich diet and 30% with the protein or unsaturated fat diet.

If you are a *vegan* and still wish to try this diet program, you have to accept the fact that it will be more difficult for you and you may not be able to lose as much weight as other patients. Since vegans have to rely on legumes as the source of protein leading to a higher daily carbohydrate consumption. They cannot stay with Phase 1 straightly. The vegan diet is low in vitamin B and iron. Daily dietary supplement is needed. Of all the legumes, soy protein has the best protein type and the lowest amount of carbohydrates. Vegan will be allowed to consume soy products during Phase 1. However, you have to watch out for the sodium and fat contents of these soy products. Another product that is suitable for vegan dieters is called Textured Soy Protein (TSP). It is made from soybeans but with the soybean oil removed by a natural process. Natural peanut butter is usually high in fat. However, there is a new peanut protein powder that has the peanut oil removed by a natural process. This becomes a good source of protein for the vegan dieters.

- *How much should you eat?* You should eat enough to stop your hunger. Remember that you will feel fuller an hour or two after a protein meal. Remember you can eat or snack every 3 to 4 hours. A rule of thumb is not to eat protein that is bigger than your palm at each setting and your bowl of vegetables should not be bigger than your protein. If you are still hungry after this, eat some more. Just do not overeat. Remember the term *glycemic load* we discussed in chapter 11? Even when you eat vegetables with a low glycemic index, the glycemic load is determined by the portion size. You can eat again later when you are hungry later. Although you do not have to count calories on this diet, you cannot expect to lose weight if you eat one turkey per day. Unlike what your mother told you, you do not have to finish all the food on your plate. Save it and eat it later when you are hungry. There is no limit as to the time of the day that you should stop eating. You can eat in the middle of the night if you need to. Some diets do not want you to eat after 6 o'clock because you may not be able to burn off the carbohydrates from your meal when you go to bed. This diet is low in carbohydrates; hence, you do not need to rely on muscle activity to burn off the carbohydrates in your meal before you go to bed.

- *Jell-O Light® or Juicy Gels® for desert.* You may add a small amount of sugar free whipped cream that you whip yourself using a light whipping cream and Splenda®, or a small amount of table cream to improve the flavor.

- *Drink plenty of water per day.* It helps your kidneys to get rid of the by-products of lipolysis (fat burning), namely ketones. Ketones are forms of fuel released from fat when fat is changed into fatty acids and glycerol. Fatty acids change into energy and ketones. Glycerol changes into energy and glucose (glucogenesis). Only the brain, heart and kidney cells can use ketone as fuel effectively. If you allow the ketones to accumulate in your tissues, you might experience muscle aches, headaches, bad breath, abdominal cramps and loss of appetite (a good side effect). By drinking more water, ketones can be eliminated from the body by the kidneys more effectively. Since ketones carry a certain number of calories, you are actually excreting calories in the urine by eliminating ketone out of your body! Decaffeinated tea or coffee, Crystal Light®, caffeine free diet soft drinks, and low-sodium homemade soups are allowed and can be *included* in your daily water consumption calculation. Green tea might be able to help to burn off some calories. It contains theanine, which is an amino acid, which helps with relaxation. Green tea contains polyphenols that have demonstrated antioxidant and anti-cancer properties. Table 33 gives you an estimate as to how much you should be drinking per day. Do not over-drink. The quantity is related to your body weight. Observe the color of your urine. It should be very light yellow in color. If the color gets darker then you are not drinking enough fluid.

Table 33. Suggested Maximum Daily Fluid Intake.

Body Weight (lb.)	Suggested Maximum Fluid Intake (ml)	Maximum Number of 8 oz Glass
120	1650	7
140	1900	8
160	2150	9
180	2400	10
200	2620	11
220	2820	12
240	3000	13
260	3170	14
280	3330	14
300	3450	15
320	3600	15
340	3740	16

If you have a large number of ketones in the urine, your fluid requirement will also increase. It is because ketones draw an extra amount of body water into the urine as the ketones get excreted. However, do not over drink because it can result in water intoxication. Significant sodium and potassium loss can result in over hydration that causes muscle weakness and cardiac arrhythmias. A simple blood test can identify this deficiency.

Another liquid you can have is clear consommé. Low-sodium chicken or beef or vegetable consommés (diluted with water) are all very good if you are not on a potassium restricted diet. There are regular bouillon cubes that are commercially available but they are higher in sodium content and are not suitable for hypertensive patients. Low-sodium bouillon cubes can be purchased in health food store. You need to learn to read labels. The percent of body water is different in males and females because of the difference in the percentage of body fat. To have good hydration, males should have at least 60% of their body weight as water, and females should have more than 50%.

Water loss during dieting is due to:

1. A decreased insulin level leads to decrease in insulin-mediated renal tubular sodium reabsorption. Therefore, extracellular and intravascular volumes decrease

2. Utilization of glycogen, 3 to 4 g of water per g of glycogen

3. Utilization of muscle, 19 to 25 g of water per g of nitrogen

4. Utilization of fat, 10 to 15% of fat is water

- *Watch the sodium content in food and drinks.* Patients often tell me that they do not eat a high salt diet because they do not add, or add a very little amount of salt to their cooking. This does not guarantee that they are on a low salt diet. The Canada Food Guide for

Healthy Eating allows 2200 mg of sodium per day. Americans consume 4000 mg daily and Canadians consume 3200 mg. Please note that the 2200 mg of sodium is what you are "allowed" to take in everyday. It is not the minimum requirement. In order to replace the body's average daily sodium loss, the body only needs 550 mg of sodium per day. Half a teaspoon of regular table salt is about 1000 mg of sodium. It is extremely hard to count the total amount of sodium that you have consumed per day. It is because all living things contain sodium, even lettuce, meat, bread etc. The rule of thumb is to make sure the sodium content of your food item is less than 170 mg of sodium per serving. What about a food item that contains 220 mg of sodium? You can still eat it as long as you do not eat more than 1 serving and you drink more fluid to force the kidneys to force it out of your body.

FAQ

- *What can I have for breakfast?* You can have anything that you are allowed to eat at any time of the day. No one ever said that you have to have eggs for breakfast. A study done at the University of California found that the consumption of two boiled eggs daily did not increase cholesterol levels. Researchers from the Harvard School of Public Health found no significant correlation between egg consumption and cardiovascular disease in healthy individuals. The study, published in the Journal of the American Medical Association, also found no difference in cholesterol levels between those who ate less than one egg a week and those who ate more than one egg a day. If in doubt, eat only the egg white that has zero cholesterol. Patients sometimes have home made soup, or chicken. You will have more variety when you advance to Phase 2. There is no limit on the time of the day that you can eat. There is such a thing as an "all day breakfast", where you can have "steak and egg" for breakfast. Who said that you could not have chicken for breakfast? There is no such thing as breakfast dog food, lunch dog food or dinner dog food. Food is food. Commonly consumed food for breakfast are egg white omelets, hard boil eggs, vegetable soup with meat, protein shakes, cookies or biscotti with coffee or tea, SMAPS cereal with coffee or protein shake, a piece of grilled chicken breast, Bran Crispbread with coffee or protein shake and very low-carb flexseed bread.

- *Do calories count?* The simplest answer is yes. You cannot expect to eat a whole turkey per day and expect to lose weight. However, one calorie from sugar is not equal to one calorie from meat. The calorie from sugar promotes insulin secretion whereas the one from meat does not. This is why you can eat a 1500 calories diet that is low in carbohydrate and still lose weight. The same number of calories in a high-carbohydrate diet will cause weight gain. If you rely on calorie counting only, you usually have to eat 1/3 less food per day to lose 1 pound per week. This is not very efficient. It makes sense that the less you eat, the more weight you can lose. However, if your calorie intake is very low, the body will try to slow down your metabolism to compensate for the lack of energy intake. This is why people on a very low calorie diet lose hair. Their hair will come back once they increase their protein and calorie intake.

- *Can I eat Protein Bars?* Things like protein bars may sound like a good idea, but it is best to stay away from them and other pre-packaged "convenience" foods at least until Phase 2. These products have high amounts of sugar alcohol. They want you to believe that sugar alcohol does not affect your weight. Some bars have glycerin which, while not a carbohydrate, has been known to stall the fat burning process. In addition, there are a lot of bad fats (saturated fat) in some of those bars. There are protein shakes that are made from egg, whey and/or soy protein isolates. Some of them may not contain all the essential amino acids that you require daily. Occasional use is allowed, but not more than once a day

- *I cheated last night when I ate out, what can I do?* Do not panic. Nobody is perfect and we all have weak moments. Jump right back on the diet as soon as possible. You should never let one indiscretion lead you back to a lifetime of destructive eating. Sure, your weight loss will be slowed down but so what? You are in it for the long haul. The carbohydrate that you indulged in will not be stored as fat as yet. It will be stored in the form of glycogen and deposited in the muscles and liver. When you store glycogen, you will also retain some water. Hence, the weight gain looks worse than it actually is. Your job is to get back on track and use up the glycogen in the next two to three days. If you give up and eat more carbohydrates the next meal, then you will gain fat weight.

- *Should my children go on this diet?* There has been a three-fold increase in obesity amongst children in Canada in the past decade. Diseases associated with obesity in children are also on the rise. Hence, it is important for children to get counseling before it is too late. We have to re-educate parents, doctors and teachers as to what is considered as junk food so that they can, in turn, teach our children to eat healthily.

- *Can I eat sugar free candy or popsicles?* Occasional use is fine but we prefer that you use it sparingly. Diet candies and popsicles contain high levels of sugar alcohols. Too much sugar alcohols can cause diarrhea or lessen your ability to burn fat. Some patients can also respond to the sweetness of the sweetener and increase insulin secretion. Sugar alcohols also carry calories, even though they are lower than in real sugar. For people who eat large portions, the extra calories from the sugar alcohol will count.

- *Your diet is low on fruits; will I be deficient in vitamins?* You will be eating all kinds of green and leafy vegetables and they are full of vitamins. Fruits that are rich in vitamins will be reintroduced to your diet once you are on Phase 2. Sharks, lions and tigers do not eat fruits and they obtain their vitamins from fish and meat. This is called the food chain. Nutrients transfer from one animal to another animal. If in doubt, you can take a multi-vitamin

- *Is caffeine allowed in this diet?* It is allowed if you do not have any counter-indications for taking caffeine, such as insomnia, gastro-intestinal reflux disease, palpitations, and an anxiety disorder. However, caffeine drinks have diuretic effects if they are over consumed. Then there are studies that show caffeine intake is associated with increased thermogenesis and fat burning. Ingestion of caffeine can increase the basal metabolic rate by 10 to 30% for 1 to 3 hours[3-5]. However, this effect is short lived. The patient has to take in enough caffeine every 3 to 4 hours to sustain this fat burning effect. High doses of caffeine may produce fine tremors of the extremities, which can lead to weight loss. In order to help you to lose weight, you should not add sugar, milk, or cream to your coffee or tea. You can also increase your thermogenesis by keeping the room cool and not compensating by wearing more clothing. Most of these studies were done with caffeine pills and not with coffee or tea[5]. Hence, the effect of caffeinated coffee on water balance is still controversial. Chronic coffee drinkers are not at risk of high blood pressure. People who seldom drink coffee can experience a rise of high blood pressure for 2-3 hours after consumption. Drinking more than 3 cups of caffeine per day without an adequate amount of calcium per day will lead to bone loss. Make sure to take calcium supplements when needed.

- *You have written "no bread", can I eat whole-wheat bread or 7-grain bread?* Similar questions were asked about Quinoa. Patients very frequently asked me if they could eat a "high-protein grain" called Quinoa. They use the term "high protein" very loosely. When you call a food item high-protein, protein should be the main macro-nutrient. A quarter cup of cooked Quinoa weighs 42g. There is 2.5g of fat, 29.3g of carbohydrate (2.5g of fiber and 26.8g of net-carb), and 5.6g of protein only. Carbohydrate is therefore the main macro-nutrient, not protein. Hence, you cannot call Quinoa a high protein grain product. It is a carbohydrate product with some protein in it. Quinoa may be higher in protein content than other grain products; however, because of the high carbohydrate content, it is not suitable for this diet program. You maybe able to find low-carb bread that contains only 1 g of net-carb per slice and is suitalbe for this phase 1 diet. However it is no readily available in ordinary grocery stores. Try to locate specialty store such as OntarioNutiriton.ca on the internet.

	Total Carb (g)	Fiber (g)	Net-carb (g)		Equivalent in sugar (tsp)
			Sugar	Starch	
7-Grain	12.1	1.7	2.6	7.8	2.6
Whole-Wheat	12.9	1.9	1.6	9.4	2.8
White	12.7	0.6	1.1	11.0	3.0
Pumpernickel	15.2	2.1	0.2	12.9	3.2
Rye	15.5	1.9	1.2	14.4	3.9

Table 34. Carbohydrate Content of Different Types of Bread (Per Slice)[6].

- *"I cannot eat like this for the rest of my life."* The Phase 1 diet is only for a short period of time. As you used up all your glycogen storage from the muscles and liver, you will start to burn fat as the main source of energy production. At that time, you will be switched to Phase 2 diet. You will be given the Phase 3 diet plan (maintenance phase) if you are going away for business or holidays. You will lose the most weight on Phase 1.

References:

1. Poon P, Poon D, Wong M, Endogenous Insulin Production in Obese NIDDM Patients taking Insulin. Obesity Oct 2008;16 supplement 1:S251.

2. Toschke AM, Kuchenhoff H, Koletzko B. Meal Frequency and Childhood Obesity. Obesity Research 2005;11:1932-8.

3. Astrup A, et al. Caffeine: a double blind, placebo-controlled study of its thermogenic, metabolic, and cardiovascular effects in healthy volunteers. Am J Clin Nutr 1990;51:759-67.

4. Dulloo AG, et al. Normal caffeine consumption: influence on thermogenesis and daily energy expenditure in lean and post obese human volunteers. Am J Clin Nutr 1989;49:44-50.

5. Bracci D, et al. Effects of caffeine on energy metabolism, heart rate, and methylxanthine metabolism in lean and obese women. Am J Physiol 1995;E:671-8.

6. USDA National Nutrient Database for Standard Reference, release 18, October 2005.

"Medication may treat the number,
Weight loss treats the cause."

18: PHASE TWO
CONTINUED WEIGHT LOSING PHASE

If you fail to lose a minimum of 7 to 10 pounds during the first two weeks and if you do not have a urine ketone level of greater than 1.5 mmol/L (15 mg/dL), then you have not been following the diet plan correctly (either knowingly or unknowingly). You are not ready to advance to Phase 2 yet. Most of the time it is because you have "hidden" carbohydrates and salt in your diet without being aware if it. We will ask you to log all foods and drinks you have had for one week and we will go over them with you carefully. There are times when you are unable to go into ketosis because of the types of medication you are taking. You will be staying in the induction phase for more than the usual two weeks. It is not harmful to stay on the induction phase as long as you do not find the limited food selection too boring; or if there is an excess of ketones in the urine. If you have a lot of weight to lose, we suggest that you stay with the induction phase for a longer period of time regardless. Make sure you are not eating too much of the non-green, non-leafy vegetables. The limit is a maximum of four cups per day. Remember that most vegetables contain absorbable carbohydrates. Over-eating them may hinder your ability to burn fat. We suggest that you increase the protein intake and cut down on the vegetables. Are you overeating?

If our body composition analyzer shows that you are losing a lot of fat weight and yet there are no ketones in the fasting urine sample, we will check for ketones in the afternoon sample also. Very often you can find ketones in the afternoon urine sample proving that you can burn fat when you are active doing your activities of daily living. It is just that you are not burning a lot of fat during sleep. Continue to stay with Phase 1 and the ketones will appear in the overnight sample also. Sometimes if you drink a lot of water during the nighttime, you are diluting the ketones in the urine sample and the concentration is too low to be detected by our chemical dipstick testing. Ketosis is not a must in our diet. If you were able to lose fat weight as indicated by our analyzer or if you were losing inches from the abdomen, you are doing fine.

If you are able to meet the above requirements, you may proceed to Phase 2 of the diet. Now your body is burning fat 24 hours a day because you have managed to decrease your insulin release by eating a low-carbohydrate diet. You can lose more weight and/or inches without being as stringent as in the fat burning Induction Phase (Phase 1). The type of new food that will be re-introduced into your diet will depend on the amount of weight that you lose in the first two weeks and the amount of ketones you produced during sleep.

The average weight loss in Phase 2 of the diet is 1.5 pounds per week or 10% of the patient's weight in 8 weeks. This amount increases with exercise. We expect your fasting urine ketone level to be greater than 0.5 mmol/L, even with an increase in carbohydrate intake. Once you have achieved this goal, we will increase your carbohydrate intake accordingly. You will still be eating foods with a relatively low carbohydrate content, low glycemic load and high in essential fatty acids and vitamins. As long as you are able to lose 1.5 pounds per week and show that you are burning fat, we will reintroduce more variety in your meals. However, if this target is not met, no new food will be introduced. If you gain weight instead of losing, we will take away the newly added foods and you will have to go back to Phase 1.

We are going to show you which additional foods you can eat during this phase. The amount of carbohydrate will be increased from 20 g in Phase 1 to 30 - 60 g depending on your progress and your amount of activity. *Keep drinking water and low-sodium low-carbohydrate fluids until the urine is very pale yellow.* If you develop muscle weakness or cramp, see your doctor and check your serum electrolytes.

Objectives of Phase 2 Diet

- To continue losing fat and water weight (average of 10% weight loss in 8 weeks)

- To start eating more carbohydrates (30 to 60 g per day), each serving should be less than 5 to 8 g of net-carb and less than 10 g of sugar alcohols (Table 24)

- To continue eating low-fat (less than 6 g of total fat and less than 2 g of saturated fat per serving) and low-salt (less than 170-200 mg of sodium per serving)

- To start exercising (150 minutes of cardiovascular exercises and some toning exercises)

- To maintain or to gain lean muscle mass

- To learn more about label reading

- To learn how to adjust your lifestyle in different social situations

- To learn stress management

- To reach normal a BMI and percent body fat

- To improve your health

List#1: Foods that you can *eat as much as you desire* and you can eat them *anytime of the day*:

- Any type of meat, including red, dark and white meats. They have to be *extra-lean* when you consume them. When possible, remove the fat and skin before or after cooking,. Ground meats from beef, chicken or turkey have to be the extra-lean variety (<10% fat). Regular ground beef is 30% fat and lean ground beef is 17% fat

- *Low-sodium* fat-free chicken or turkey breast deli meat. They can be difficult to find. They are not pre-packaged and you have to ask the worker at the deli counter if the supermarket is carrying this kind of product. Do not just go for fat-free deli meats because they are usually very high in sodium

- Any kind of fish, including the fatty type since it contains essential fatty acids. Fish has to be either fresh or frozen without added salt

- Scallops. They have very little fat and cholesterol

- Egg whites. They are pure protein without salt, fat, cholesterol and carbohydrate. It has the best amount of quality protein out of all protein sources

- Green leafy vegetables. As long as it is green in color and is the leafy part, you can have it. There are too many to list individually. Go to the supermarket and find it yourself. Cabbage is allowed but not brussel sprouts because it is higher in carbohydrates

- Olive oil and canola oil. These oils have high amounts of monounsaturated fatty acids (60%) and better omega-3 to omega-6 ratios (2 to 1) when compared to other vegetable oils

- Any kind of sweetener. Splenda® is preferred because you can cook or bake with it. You can also use stevia, a natural sweetener that has recently been approved by the FDA to use in food products

- Diet drinks, including pop, Crystal Light®, diet iced tea, coffee, black tea, herbal tea and green tea. Try to chose the types with low sodium and low caffeine contents

- Jell-O Light® jelly or similar products (not the Jell-O pudding)

- Calorie-free fruit spread but not "No sugar added" jam

- Shirataki® noodles or Tofu Shirataki® noodles. They are mainly fiber and contain minimal amounts of sugar and starch

- Low-sodium vegetable broth or bouillon, low-sodium chicken or beef broth

- Spices and herbs, as long as they do not contain salt. For example, Mrs. Dash®, McCormick® Spices, black pepper, white pepper, paprika and curry powder etc.

- Xanthan gum or guar gum (to make gravy and to thicken soup, see our cookbook for more detail)

- Vinegar, any kind

List#2: Foods that you can *eat some* daily:

- Bran Crispbread®, 2 pieces three times per day

- Very low-carb Flaxseed Bread with 1 gram of net-carb. One slice twice a day

- Shellfish. 1 small lobster tail, 5 large headless shrimps

- Egg yolk. 1 per day, if you do not have a cholesterol problem

- Calorie-free dressings. 1 tsp per serving

- Calorie-free BBQ sauce. 1 tsp per serving

- Joknal® hot sauce, mint sauce, ketchup. 1 tsp per serving

- Table cream 5-10% or soy creamer or milk. 5 ml (1 tsp) per regular cup of coffee or tea

- Sugar-free gum, candy, gummy bear, marshmallow and chocolate (such as Heart Chocolate™ with CMX®, 1 piece three times per day). Limit to *10 g* of sugar alcohols per serving. You can have 1 serving every 5 hours. Try to pick the kind that is also fat-free.

- Other fresh vegetables. A total of not more than four cups of artichoke hearts, asparagus, cauliflower, carrots, celery, cucumber, mushrooms, all kinds of bell peppers, onions, green onions, broccoli, green (string) beans, wax beans, zucchini, bean spouts, orka, pumkin, squash (avoid butternut or acorn squash), snow peas, tomatoes, cherry tomatoes, turnips, Daikon (Chinese radish), bamboo shoots, black wood ear (wood fungus), winter melon, eggplant per day. You do not have to measure them. We want you to know that these vegetables have higher carbohydrate contents than green leafy vegetables, hence it is not all you can eat

- Ginger, lemon, lime and garlic for cooking

- Low-sodium soy sauce and Half Salt® to taste

- Canned fish. Has to be "Low sodium in water" tuna or salmon. Not more than 2 cans total per week

- Tofu (bean curd) and its products (soy beans), 1 serving

- Humus or chick peas, 2 tablespoons

- Half an oz of Sesame seeds, or sunflower seeds (shelled), or pumpkin seeds (shelled)

- Sugar-free fat-free Popsicle or Freezies, 2 per serving

- Low-fat or ultra low-fat cream cheese or sour cream, 2 tablespoons

- Light or ultra light mayonnaise, 2 tablespoons

- Low-fat and trans-fat free margarine, 2 teaspoons

- Protein shakes. The best type of protein shake comes from egg protein. Do not use it more than once a day

- SMAPS® cereal. Half a cup of this cereal contains 2 net-carbohydrates

- Very low-carb Flexseed Bread. One slice twice a day

List#3: You may eat a maximum of two of the following items per day:

DO NOT EAT MORE THAN TWO ITEMS

- Half of a Kiwi, or orange, or grapefruit

- Half a cup of Cantaloupe, or Honeydew, or Watermelon, or Plum, or berries

- Cherries - 5 to 10

- Fat-free low-carbohydrate yogurt - 1serving, e.g. Source®, Silhouette®, Astro®

- Fat-free and low-sodium cottage cheese, ½ cup

- Low-fat and low-sodium cheese, 1 oz

- Rice cake, 1

- Sugar-free Creamsicle or Fudgsicle. 1 per serving

- Low-carbohydrate bread products, has to be less than 7 g of net-carb per slice, e.g. High-protein Pita, Mama Lupa Wrap®, Joseph's ® Lavash Bread (pita), Weight Watcher's® whole-wheat bread (available at most grocery stores)

- Low-carbohydrate low-fat muffin or pancake, less than 7 g of net-carb per serving, e.g. Dixie Dinners' Muffin mix

- Low-carbohydrate cereal products, 1 serving, e.g. Hi-Lo cereal®, Dixie Diners' Hot Cereal®, Fiber 1 cereal® (available at most grocery stores). Fiber 1 cereal® contains the highest amount of net-carb (11 g) among all these three cereals

- Milk, skim or 1%, ½ cup to 1 cup per day to be used in your cereal, tea or coffee

- Soy milk, unsweetened unflavored soy milk, net-carb of 2 to 4 g per serving, 1 cup

- Nuts, unsalted - macadamia (5 whole), almond (10 whole), walnut (6 halves), pecan (6 halves), Cashew (10 whole), or peanut (12 whole), avoid chestnut

- Skinni™ Spaghetti, 2 oz dry weight

- Low-carb Low-fat cracker, e.g. Shibolim® Crisp Snax, 7 pieces

- Low-carb Blended Ice Vanilla Latte, e.g. Big Train®, 1 serving

- Bowel Buddy® Bran Wafers (combat constipation), 2 cookies

- Low sodium Roasted Soybeans, e.g. Dixie Diners' Soy Beanits™

- Russell Stover® Sugar Free snack bar, 1

- Atkins™ Endulge Peanut Caramel Cluster Bar, 1

- Alcohol, 4 oz of wine, or 1 oz of hard liquor, or 8 oz of low-carb beer

- Oatmeal, 1 cup cooked (do not use the instant type of oatmeal because of its high sodium content, use this not more than once a week because it is high in net-carb)

- Popcorn (low fat and low sodium), may use a buttery flavored spray to enhance the taste, 2 cups popped

- Beef jerky or soy jerky, low-sodium type, 1 serving

- Pork rinds, 1 serving (avoid if you have excessive water retention or high blood pressure)

Remind yourself not to eat all the allowed carbohydrates in one sitting. Start adding more variety to the vegetables in your diet. We do not want you to eat more vegetables in quantity, but you can have vegetables that are higher in carbohydrate content now. You are allowed to pick *two* of the above items per day, but try to eat them separately. For example, try not to eat fruit with nuts at the same time. Note that there are quantity limitations on some of the items since they are full of carbohydrates. Please be aware that most cheeses have carbohydrates, saturated fat and salt. Read the food label carefully. Most shellfish also has some carbohydrate. Crab is the exception. Raw oysters are at the other extreme containing about 1.4 g of carbohydrate per 30 g. Organ meats (such as liver) also contain some carbohydrate and a certain amount of unsaturated fat, therefore we prefer you to eat them only occasionally.

A small amount of nuts is allowed. However, please pay attention to the quantity. Nuts are full of fat and carry a lot of calories (Table 32). The

Table 35. Nutritional Information of Twelve Grams of Dry Roasted Unsalted Nuts.

	Almond (10 whole)	Walnut (6 halves)	Macadamia (5 whole)	Pecan (8 halves)	Cashew (10 whole)	Peanut (12 whole)
Calories	70	80	87	90	81	72
Protein	2.6	1.9	0.9	1.2	2.7	2.9
Fat	6.1	7.9	9.1	9	6.6	6
Poly-	1.5	5.7	0.2	2.5	1.1	1.9
Mono-	3.9	1.1	7.2	5.3	3.9	2.9
Sat-	0.5	0.7	1.5	0.7	1.3	0.8
Chole.	0	0	0	0	0	0
Carb.	2.4	1.7	1.6	1.6	4.6	2.6
Fiber-	1.0	0.8	1.0	1.1	0.4	1.2

good thing about nut is that its fat is of the polyunsaturated and monounsaturated type. Most of them have very little of carbohydrates except cashew. Only the dry roasted unsalted nuts are allowed.

Once you have started to burn fat, you should think of limiting the amount of "bad" fat in your diet. You were told to use cream for your coffee or tea during the Induction Phase because it has fewer carbohydrates than milk. Since you are allowed to have more carbohydrates in the Continued Weight Losing Phase, it is safe to switch back to skim or 1% milk, especially if you have high cholesterol or coronary heart disease. Dietary plant sterols (plant cholesterol), especially sitostanol, reduce serum cholesterol by inhibiting cholesterol absorption[1]. Sometimes a patient may notice that the rate of weight loss varies from week to week even though the patient has been eating the same type and quantity of food. This is particularly true in female patients. It can be due to *water retention*. Avoid foods with high sodium contents such as processed meat, cheese, canned food, sauces, or pickled food. Use a potassium based salt instead (Chapter 14).

Table 36. Sodium Content of Commonly Consumed Foods.

Antacid in water	564 mg
Apple pie (1/8 frozen)	208 mg
Bacon (4 slices)	548 mg
Bagel (1)	245 mg
Beef jerky (1 large piece)	438 mg
Big Mac, (1)	1050 mg
Bread, Italian (1 slice)	176 mg
Cheese, Cheddar (1 cup)	701 mg
Cheese, cottage (1 cup)	911 mg
Cheese, cream, fat free (1 tbsp.)	85 mg
Cheese, Parmesan (1 cup)	1861 mg
Chicken pie (frozen)	907 mg
Chicken dinner (fast food)	2243 mg
Chicken breast (3 oz)	64 mg
Chicken noodle soup (1 can)	1106 mg
Chicken Caesar salad with dressing	2625 mg
Corn flakes (1 cup)	256 mg
Cola, with saccharin	75 mg
Cola, regular	126 mg
Corned beef (3 oz)	802 mg
Dill pickle	928 mg
Dry milk (1/2 cup)	322 mg
English muffin	293 mg
Ham (3 oz)	1114 mg
Hot dog (1)	504 mg
Instant mashed potato	485 mg
Jumbo burger (fast food)	990 mg
Ketchup (1 tbsp.)	156 mg
Lima beans, canned (1 cup)	809 mg
Macaroni and cheese (1 cup)	1058 mg

Table 36. Sodium Content of Commonly Consumed Foods (continued).

Meat loaf (frozen dinner)	1304 mg
Milk (1 cup)	122 mg
Mixed veggies, frozen (1 cup)	64 mg
Mixed veggies, canned (1 cup)	243 mg
Mushrooms, canned (1 cup)	663 mg
Peas, green, canned (1 cup)	428 mg
Peas, green, frozen (1 cup)	115 mg
Pork grind (1 oz)	521 mg
Potato chips (10)	200 mg
Pretzels, hard plain, salted (10)	1029 mg
Salami (2 slices)	607 mg
Salmon, baked (3 oz)	55 mg
Salmon, pink, canned (3 oz)	470 mg
Salmon, smoked (3 oz)	1700 mg
Salt (1 tsp)	1938 mg
Sauerkraut (1 cup)	1560 mg
Soup, chicken veggie, canned (1 cup)	1068 mg
Soup, onion mix, dry form (1 package)	3493 mg
Sour cream (1 cup)	123 mg
Soy Sauce (1 tsp)	1029 mg
Spaghetti sauce (1 cup)	1030 mg
Sunflower seeds, dry roasted (1/4 cup)	250 mg
Steak, Sirloin (3 oz)	53 mg
Tomato soup (1 cup)	932 mg
Tomato sauce (1 cup)	1498 mg
Tuna, canned (3oz)	387 mg
Vegetable juice (1 cup)	883 mg
Wendy's spicy chicken fillet sandwich	1480 mg
Whopper with cheese (1)	1450 mg

(Source: U.S. Department of Agriculture)

The recommended sodium allowance is below 2400 mg per day. The WHO recommends 1700 mg per day for people with hypertension. The average North American daily sodium intake is approx. 4000 mg per day! The average Canadian's is about 3400 mg per day. Do you know that our daily sodium requirement to stay healthy is only 550 mg per day?

The amount of female hormone varies with the phase of a woman's menstrual cycle. At the middle of the cycle, just before ovulation, estrogen level is at its peak. A high estrogen level promotes energy, creativity and libido. Immediately after ovulation, the egg starts to manufacture progesterone, which promotes relaxation. A few days before menstrual bleeding, both the estrogen and progesterone are at the lowest levels. This may cause *Premenstrual Syndrome*. The body and mind are more sensitive to all forms of stress. It may also cause excessive fluctuations in blood glucose levels and fluid retention. Some women get very strong cravings for starch and sugar.

The amounts of exercise or activity, the temperature outside and some types of medication (arthritis medications, Alka-Seltzer, oral fleet, fleet enema) have some bearing on the amount of water retention. Another possible factor is constipation. Even if there is no weight loss when you step on the scale, you may still be losing inches since your body is burning fat, as shown by the presence of ketones in the urine. There is no need to be discouraged. We will help you to analyze the cause of your water retention and adjust accordingly. Simply drinking more water or decreasing the amount of table salt used may solve the problem. If it is due to pre-menstrual bloating, the problem will correct itself once your period is finished. Another common reason for swollen extremities is medication (Chapter 10). Your doctor may have to adjust your medication accordingly.

At this time in your dieting, you should look into exercising to increase your metabolism (Chapter 13). In addition, you may need to use dietary supplements to help you lose weight and maintain good health (Chapter 14). The most important one is calcium since this diet is low in dairy products in Phase 1 and ketosis can lead to calcium loss. However, don't think that dairy products are the only source of calcium. Calcium is plentiful in vegetables and proteins. With ketosis, a certain amount of calcium will be lost in the urine that requires replacement. For a patient who is diabetic, hypertensive or has coronary artery disease, magnesium supplementation is indicated. You can purchase a combination pill that contains a mixture of calcium, magnesium and vitamin D and take it daily. A patient who takes cholesterol-lowering medication (statin) should take Co-enzyme Q10, 30-60 mg daily.

By the end of two months on this diet, you should have lost at least ten percent of your weight. Most diet experts consider losing ten percent of your weight as a major milestone. You will feel lighter, more energetic, and be able to fit into clothing that was too tight before. People will notice your weight loss and pay you compliments. You can stay on this diet until you lose fifteen, twenty, or thirty percent of excess weight. Another set of blood work should be done to check your blood glucose, cholesterol, triglycerides, and liver and kidney functions. Your Body Mass Index and Percentage of Body Fat will be re-calculated.

Your goal is to continue to lose weight until your Body Mass Index is below 27 and/or Percentage of Body Fat is below 22% for men and 34% for women. The ideal Body Mass Index is 23 (19 to 25 is the normal range), and the ideal Percentage of Body Fat is shown in table 35.

Table 37. Ideal Body Fat Ranges.		
Female	20 to 39 years old	21% to 33%
	40 to 59 years old	23% to 34%
	60 to 79 years old	24% to 36%
Male	20 to 39 years old	8% to 20%
	40 to 59 years old	11% to 22%
	60 to 79 years old	13% to 25%

Some weeks you may find that you did not lose very much weight. However, if your waistline continues to trim, it may mean that you are losing fat and/or gaining some muscles (from eating more protein and doing more weight training exercises), and/or retaining water.

Your weight gain did not happen overnight, so weight loss cannot occur overnight. The occasional slip-up on the diet does happen. Do not give up. Work harder the next day to make up for the mistake. Go back to the Phase 1 diet for 3 days and it will work again. Unlike the calorie-counting diet, there is no plateau on this diet. You will continue to lose weight until your goal is met. If you were able to lose more than 1.5 pounds per week and demonstrated ketones in the urine, you can pick 3 items from the Phase 2 shopping list. We have patients who eat 4 items from the list and still lose 1.5 pounds of fat every week. In general, the more active you are, the more carbohydrates you will be able to tolerate. Exercise will increase your metabolism. The reverse is true; if you are having difficulty in losing weight in Phase 2, you may pick only 1 item per day instead of 2 until your situation changes. We have mentioned before that certain medications can slow down your metabolism. You might have fractured your ankle and are now wearing a cast, or you might be suffering from severe low back pain and are now bed ridden. During these situations of inactivity, you may not be able to tolerate as much carbohydrate as before.

Table 38 shows you some of the common reasons why patients are unable to lose weight on this phase of the diet. Sometimes patients recall only those things they are supposed to eat and forget that they had cheated. A food diary will be helpful. This also makes the patients more aware of the food choices that they are making.

Table 38. Pitfalls of Phase Two Diet and Their Remedies.

Causes of failure	Remedies
Cheating (knowingly or unknowingly)	Food diary. Return to Phase 1 if you gain weight
Exceeding the limits on Phase 2 selections (e.g. eating more than 2 items per day, or over eating the amount allowed per item)	Adhere to the quantity allowed
Water retention	If it is due to premenstrual retention, the problem will correct itself. Lower salt intake and drink more water Side effects of medications - see if physician can adjust Decrease amount of carbohydrates if consuming excess amounts
Muscle gain	Self-limiting

Top 10 Excuses for Cheating

10. Holiday

9. Too many parties

8. My birthday, or my friend's birthday

7. I have to cook for my family

6. I was told to have a banana everyday

5. The label on the pill bottle said that I have to have a banana everyday

4. They said that I have to eat carbohydrates everyday, otherwise my brain will not be able to function

3. Too much stress

2. They make me eat it

1. "I did not cheat"

RECIPES FOR THE CONTINUED WEIGHT LOSS PHASE

THE COMPLETE MEAL

"The Complete Meal" contains protein, fiber, fat and vitamins. Yet it is low in carbohydrate and sodium. You should make a big pot of this and eat this soup any time you like. You may alter the ingredients to suit your taste. The recipe calls for:

- Cubes of lean beef, turkey, or chicken, carrots, green cabbage, green beans, mushrooms, zucchini, minced garlic cloves, tomato paste, dried basil and oregano for flavor, low sodium vegetable broth, and olive oil

- Brown the minced garlic in olive oil using a large pot. Sauté all the vegetables until soft

- Pour in the low sodium vegetable or chicken broth and add enough water to cover all the vegetables

- Cook until the beans and the carrots are soft

- Sauté the meat in a different skillet with garlic and olive oil until brown and put them into the soup

- Add tomato paste, basil and oregano, and simmer until done

CHICKEN AND TOFU VEGETABLE SOUP

- Buy a whole rotisserie chicken from the supermarket and separate the meat from the bone. Chop the meat into small pieces and discard the fat

- Brown three cloves of garlic and 3 small onions in ¼ cup of olive oil using a large pot

- Add ½ pound of sliced fresh mushrooms, 1 cup of diced carrots, and 1 cup of diced celery. Cook until soft

- Add 2 cans of low sodium chicken broth and 6 cans of water (or use low sodium vegetable or chicken bouillon)

- Pour in all the chicken pieces and add 1 box of soft tofu (after you have diced the tofu into small cubes)

- Put in some basil and thyme as needed

HOT POT

- This is a favorite Chinese dish. You can find all the ingredients in Chinese supermarkets

- Add low sodium chicken broth and bring it to a boil

- Add soft tofu (1/2 box), shrimps (4), clams (5), beef slices (5) and/or pork slices (5), and lettuce in small pieces (1/4 head) or other Chinese vegetables

- Do not cover the pot and do not over cook the ingredients. It only takes 1 minute to cook

- Add 1 teaspoon of olive oil and ½ teaspoon of sesame oil and serve immediately

LOW CARBOHYDRATE STEAMED EGG CUSTARD By Beckie Poon

Ingredients (single serving):

1 large egg

1 teaspoon of table cream

2 packages of Splenda®

- Add Splenda® to ½ cup of cold water

- Beat egg with fork until smooth

- Mix the two ingredients together and mix them well along with 1 teaspoon of table cream

- Sieve the mixture, refrigerate for 8 hours or overnight

- Sieve the mixture again into a glass or ceramic bowl just big enough to hold the content

- Steam in medium/low heat for 4 minutes. Lift lid for 2 seconds to let steam out. Steam for another 2 min. Lift lid again for 2 seconds and steam for another 2 min

- Serve hot or refrigerated

ROAST BEEF WRAP

Ingredients:

¼ cup of ultra-low-fat cream cheese

4 low-carb wraps

½ red onion, sliced

4 lettuce leaves

4 cucumber spears

8 oz of roast beef

- Spread cream cheese over the wrap. Lay all ingredients on top of one another. Roll up from the bottom.

ALMOND CINNAMON BALLS by Elaine Ross

The almond balls should be soft inside, with a very strong cinnamon flavor. They harden with keeping, so it is a good idea to freeze some and thaw them when required.

Ingredients:

1 ½ cups ground almonds

1/3 cup Splenda®

1 tablespoon ground cinnamon

2 egg whites

Oil for greasing

Method:

- Preheat the oven to 350 degrees F

- Oil a large baking sheet

- Mix together the ground almonds, Splenda and cinnamon

- Beat the egg whites until they begin to stiffen and fold into almond mixture to make a fairly firm mixture

- Wet your hands with cold water and roll mixture into balls. Place these on the prepared baking sheet

- Bake for about 15 minutes; so they remain slightly soft inside…too much cooking will make them hard and tough. Slide a metal spatula under the balls to release them from the baking sheet and allow to cool

- This recipe makes 15 balls. Instead of eating 10 almonds per day, you may have 5 balls per day

STIR-FRY BEEF AND VEGETABLES

Ingredients:

2 tablespoons of olive oil

8 oz of beef, sliced into small pieces

(you may substitute with chicken or seafood).

1 tablespoon of soy sauce

¼ tablespoon of sesame seed oil

1 clove of garlic, chopped

1 plate of mixed vegetables (choice of green, yellow or red peppers, celery, mushrooms, broccoli, Chinese greens, etc.) cut in small pieces

- Marinate the beef with soy sauce and sesame seed oil

- Heat up the frying pan with 1 tablespoon of olive oil. When the oil is hot, throw in the garlic

- Once the garlic is browned, pour in the marinated beef slices and stir-fry for 1 minute. Remove the beef from the frying pan

- Add another tablespoon of oil and pour in all the vegetables when the oil is hot. Stir-fry the vegetable for 2 minutes. Add 1 tablespoon of water and continue to cook with high heat

- Once the vegetables are soft, return the beef to the frying pan. Stir all the food together and serve immediately.

PORK CHOPS WITH CUMIN, COLLARD GREENS AND SPINACH

BY D.D. GADJANSKI

Ingredients:

4 pork chops

¼ teaspoon mustard seed

1 bunch collard greens

½ teaspoon ground ginger

1 bunch spinach

4 cloves garlic

3 florets of cauliflower, sliced

2 stalks celery

4 pieces green onion

- Fry pork chops with olive oil in a frying pan with salt substitute, pepper and cumin sprinkled on both sides of the pork chops

- When done, remove on to paper towel and cover

- Sauté green onions, celery, ground ginger, cauliflower and garlic. When almost done, add chopped spinach, collard greens and black pepper

- Slice pork chops into thin strips (trim off all fats)

- Place vegetable on a plate with sliced pork chops on top

- You can add a bit of apple cider vinegar to hot vegetables for additional aroma

You can find more recipes in the "Dr. Poon's Metabolic Diet Cookbook".

Reference:

1. Miettiene TA et al. Reduction of serum cholesterol with sitostanol-ester margarine in a mildly hypercholesterolemic population. New England Journal of Medicine 1995;333:1308-12.

19: PHASE THREE MAINTENANCE PHASE

If you go back to your old way of eating, you will gain back the weight. We are going to teach you to select the right food groups so that you can maintain your weight and yet enable you to have a wide variety of foods.

The Canada's Food Guide was first introduced in 1942 during the Second World War. It was meant to suggest food rations during a time of war, while endeavoring to prevent nutritional deficiencies and to improve the health of Canadians. There was a shortage of food, especially protein and milk. The guide helped people to achieve the total caloric requirement while eating a diet that was low in protein. The diet plan was not formulated by choice but by necessity. The original food guide evolved from a document called the Dietary Standard in 1939. The plan was to provide the amounts of essential nutrients considered adequate to meet the needs of practically all healthy persons. Because of the shortage of protein, the question that was posted to the experts was - what is the minimal amount of protein each person needs per day to stay healthy? This led to a food guide that is low in protein and high in carbohydrates. It had nothing to do with "healthy eating".

The Food Guide has gone through many names and many changes since. In 1992, the official name given to the food guide was Canada's Food Guide to Healthy Eating. It had a rainbow design and separated food into four food groups (six food groups in the original food guide).

It suggested that you could have 12 servings of grain products, which is equal to 12 slices of bread, or 6 cups of pasta! You could only have 150 g of meat or fish per day, which is equal to 5 oz. It was not surprising when researchers concluded from the past ten years of experience, that eating according to the Canada's Food Guide would cause *weight gain* if you did not exercise as required.

The latest one was introduced in 2007 and the new name is "Eating Well with Canada's Food Guide". It recommends more vegetables, fresh fruit, whole grains, milk and low calorie low fat food. Physical activity is deemed necessary. The guide also suggested that people over 50 years old should take vitamin D supplements. They found that they had to modify the past Food Guide to help Canadian to prevent diabetes, coronary heart disease and obesity. Note that the Food Guide is for prevention and not for treatment. This Food Guide is to help people who are healthy with normal weight and do not have to take medications to maintain their good health and weight. They never claim that this is the way to eat to treat diabetes or to promote weight lost. The Food Guide is a healthy diet for the healthy people. If you are not a healthy person, this dietary recommendation may not be the right diet for you. We would like to consider our Metabolic Diet plan as the *healthy diet for the obese.*

The Food Pyramid proposed by the FDA of the U.S. has similar guidelines regarding daily carbohydrate intake (6 to 11 servings) with limited protein and fat. In 1995, a report in the Journal of the American Dietetic Association showed that although the percentage of calories from fat in the American's diet decreased from 41% in 1958 to 34% in 1993, the prevalence of overweight U.S. adults *increased* from 23% in 1958 to 33% in 1993. Dr. Walter Willet, a professor of nutrition at the Harvard University School of Public Health stated that the Food Pyramid is flawed. He explained that the Food Pyramid claimed that all fats are bad, all complex carbohydrates are good, all protein sources offer the same nutrition quality, and dairy should be eaten in high amounts. Dr. Willet emphasizes the quality of food choices - such as white meat over red meat; whole grains over refined grains; oils high in unsaturated fat, such as many vegetable oils, over those with saturated fat; and multivitamin use. I would like to go a little further in proposing fish over animal protein; fresh over processed meat. The American Food Guide has made some changes in 2006 and is moving in the right direction.

A study was done by the Diabetes Comprehensive Care Program at the St. Michael's Hospital in Toronto in 2006 to find out how much weight reduction Type 2 diabetic patients can achieve with their program. Patients failed to achieve any weight reduction after 12 weeks of an *intense* diet program following the Canadian Diabetic Association nutrition guidelines. These patients received counseling from dietitians, social workers, pharmacists, and physical therapists. The research leader did not provide any reason for the failure[1].

Remember…

Healthy Eating ≠ Weight Reduction

Healthy Eating ≠ Sugar Control

The Maintenance Phase is a life long program that allows you to eat a vast variety of foods. However, the principle of "too much sugar and starch is bad for you" still holds. *Avoid following the Food Guide if you have a weight and health problem.* It is good for people who are of normal weight, free of medical condition, and exercise regularly. For example, the Canada Food Guide allows too much carbohydrate in the diet that is not safe for people who are diabetic.

When a man goes from normal weight to being obese, his metabolism will never return to the pre-weight gain state, even if he returns to a normal weight and loses all the weight that he gained. As he gains weight, his adipocytes get bigger in size and the pre-adipocytes will multiply to form more adipocytes to handle the extra nutrients. Hence, the total number of adipocytes increases as he gains weight. Even when he loses his weight, although the size of the adipocytes is smaller in size, the number of adipocytes remains the same. Adipose tissue is very vascular with capillaries interwoven among the adipocytes. Hence, this man has a superior absorptive state than a man that had never been obese; even if both men are the same weight. If they consume the same amount of calories and with the same percentage of carbohydrates, the man with the history of obesity may gain weight whereas the man with no history of obesity will not. Our patients will not be able to tolerate 300 g of carbohydrate per day, as allowed by the Food Guide, even during the maintenance phase without taking the risk of regaining fat.

Objectives of Phase 3 Diet

- To maintain your weight and health

- To avoid regaining the weight you lost

- To allow you to take a break form Phase 1 or 2 during holidays or other occasions

- To allow you to have more variety of foods

- To keep the net carbohydrate below 10 g per serving and not more than 120 g per day

- To keep the glycemic load to below 5 per serving

Follow a few Simple Rules

- Foods you should avoid for the rest of your life are refined sugars, dried fruits, bleached flours, and potatoes etc (Table 40). These are likely the cause of obesity and Type 2 diabetes

- Avoid eating your daily allowance of carbohydrates in one sitting. Spread out your carbohydrate intake through out the day to avoid a sudden rise in your blood glucose. Try not to have any carbohydrates after 7 PM

- Other than your usual low carbohydrate vegetables, you can have *4 servings of grain products per day*. One serving is equal to 1 slice of bread (prefer low-carb, whole grain, whole wheat, brown, Chapati, pumpernickel, or sourdough), 30 g of low sugar cereal (low-carb, oat, wheat or rice bran, or oatmeal), ½ of a low-carb bagel, wrap, pita or bun, ½ bowl of whole wheat pasta or ½ bowl of rice

- *One serving (1/2 cup) of fruit twice a day.* Try not to eat two servings of fruit in one sitting. Chose from the berries group, the melon group, and the citrus group. Avoid banana, grapes, pineapple, mango and apple etc. A list can be found in the Appendix

- *One serving of milk product per day.* One serving equals 1 cup (250 ml) of skim milk, or 50 g (2 oz) of low-fat hard cheese, or 175 g (3/4 cup) of low-fat plain yogurt (add your own fresh fruits). Watch the sodium content of different cheese products, especially with cheese and cottage cheese. Soymilk with added calcium is a good alternative to cow's milk. Avoid soymilk with added sugar. Add sugar substitute as needed. Soymilk and tofu have a very low glycemic index and load, and are excellent for this diet

- Use good fats from olive oil, canola oil and fish. They are essential for your health

- Eat some protein every time you have carbohydrates. Dr. Barry Sears, in his book "Mastering The Zone", proposed that in order to stay in the "zone" of balance, you should eat equal amounts of protein with your carbohydrates. He wants you to choose vegetables with high fiber content and fruits. The amount of protein per meal should not exceed the size of your palm in each meal. However, if you are hungry, go ahead and eat more. You should not be required to feel hungry in order to maintain your weight

- Stay within your allowable daily caloric intake

Table 39. Daily Energy Requirements (Calories).
Men = 1.4* x [10 x (weight in kg) + 900] Women = 1.4* x [7 x (weight in kg) + 800]
*Use 1.2 if you have very low activity, and use 1.6 if you are very active.

For example, if you are a male weighing 70 kg, then you multiply 70 by 10 (70 X 10 = 700), add 900 to the product (700 + 900=1600) and multiply 1600 by 1.4, to give you 2240 calories per day. This means that you can consume 2240 calories per day and you will not gain weight

- Choose food with a low glycemic index (less than 50), low carbohydrate content (less than 10 g) and low glycemic load (less than 5) - see Appendix

- Avoid empty calories like alcohol. If you have to drink, drink one glass of dry wine or liquor, but avoid regular beer

- Avoid processed food. It has too many additives and salt. Simple is better. Eat fresh produce, fruit, meat and fish

- Stay active. Even if you are not on a diet, exercise is always good for you

- Continue your vitamins and supplements for health maintenance

- Stress management. There are people who will overeat every time there is a stressful situation. Sarah Ferguson is a good example. She gained a lot of weight after her mother passed away. You have to understand that overeating cannot get rid of your problem. Seek professional help if needed. Good sleep habits are essential. Lack of sleep triggers the munchies. During stressful moments, the brain releases corticotropin-releasing hormone, triggering the stress hormones adrenaline and cortisol to mobilize carbohydrate and fat for quick energy. If cortisol level stays high for a long period of time, it promotes an increase in appetite and elevates insulin level leading to fat gain and insulin resistance

- Weigh yourself often to get feed back. Use your glucometer. If there is a sudden rise in your glucose level, you must be eating too much carbohydrate. If there is a sudden rise in your blood pressure, you may be using too much salt or not drinking enough water. You should be able to maintain your weight within three to five pounds of your lowest weight. Before you gain more than five pounds, you need to go back to Phase 1 and lose the five pounds you've gained. The first few pounds of weight gain are usually water and glycogen. It is easier to get rid of that than fat. If you gain more than five pounds, you are likely to gain fat weight and it will take longer to burn the fat off. If you gain back more than five percent of your weight, you need to come back to see us. We will go over your food choices again with you. Consistent self-monitoring of weight is a key component of a successful weight loss maintenance program[2]

- During the holiday seasons, rather than focusing on the fact that you cannot eat a lot of the food that other people can eat, focus on how you are doing something positive for yourself by sticking to the diet and improving your health

- Try not to skip meals

- Use smaller sized plates, cups and bowls. Research showed that people eat less thinking that they already had a bigger portion

Table 40. Food that has High Carbohydrate Content and/or Calories that should be Avoided in Our Diet.

Apple juice
Apricots, dried
Avocados
Banana
Beans, kidney
Bean soup
Beer
Biscuits
Carrot cake
Cheesecake
Chestnut
Cereals, sugary type
Cheddar, processed
Chicken noodle soup
Clam chowder
Cocoa, mix
Cola, regular
Chocolate chip cookie
Corn on the cob
Cranberry juice
Croissants
Danish
Doughnuts
Dried fruits
Fast foods
Fatty meats
Fruit juice
Fruit cocktail, canned
Figs, dried
French fries
Grapes
Hotdog
Imitation crabmeat
Ice cream

Icing
Macaroni and cheese
Marshmallows
Milk, Chocolate
Muffin
Nectarines
Pineapple juice
Pizza
Potato chips
Potatoes
Prunes, dried
Pudding
Raisins
Sugar
Vegetable juice
Yogurt, regular

RECIPES FOR THE MAINTENANCE PHASE

HOT OATMEAL WITH EGG (maximum of once per week)

- Boil 1 cup of water or unsweetened calcium-fortified soy milk

- Add 1 cup of Quaker Oat® (avoid the instant type of oatmeal because it may contain salt) and stir

- Add 2 teaspoons of Splenda®

- Add 2 teaspoons of 10% table cream (optional)

- Beat 1 egg (or Omega-Pro®) and slowly pour it into the oatmeal while stirring slowly

- Serve hot

THE COMPLETE MEAL WITH PASTA or WILD RICE

Follow the recipes in Phase 2 to make the soup. Prepare the whole-wheat pasta or the wild rice according to the package. Do not over cook them since over cooking the pasta increases the glycemic index. You should limit the portion of the pasta or rice to 1 cup per meal.

FROZEN LEMON DESSERT BY DIANA FEINSTEIN

Ingredients:

3 Omega-3 eggs

2 Omega-3 egg yokes

1¼ cup of Splenda®

¾ cup of lemon juice

grated rind of ½ lemon

1½ cup of Nutriwhip Light®

- In a heavy bottomed saucepan whisk together eggs, egg yolks and Splenda®. Whisk in lemon juice

- Heat over medium heat and stir until mixture thickens and comes to a boil

- Stir in grated lemon rind and cook, stirring for 2 minutes. It will be the consistency of sour cream

- Remove from heat. Cover with plastic wrap directly onto the lemon mixture and refrigerate until cold

- Beat Nutriwhip Light® until very stiff. Fold into lemon mixture

- Place in bowl and freeze until solid

- Remove dessert from freezer 20-30 minutes before serving

WHITE CABBAGE (BOK CHOY) STIR-FRY WITH EXTRA LEAN MINCED BEEF OR PORK BY D.D. GADJANSKI

Ingredients:

2 tablespoons of olive oil

4 pieces of green onion, coarsely chopped

3 celery stalks, coarsely chopped

4 slices of dry Hungarian salami, thinly julienned

1 freshly chopped ginger root

1 pound of extra-lean ground beef or pork

¾ head of white cabbage coarsely cut

- Heat olive oil in a saucepan

- Add green onion, ginger, celery, salami, and sauté until translucent

- Add minced meat

- Sauté further until meat has lost its fresh red color and starts getting cooked

- Ad the white cabbage and stir well

- Add salt substitute and pepper to taste

You can find more recipes in *"Dr. Poon's Metabolic Diet Cookbook"*.

References:

1. Jessica Bonney, Henry Halapy, Yvonne Mullan. Evaluation of a Multidisciplinary Weight Management Program for People with Type 2 Diabetes. Canadian Journal of Diabetes 2006;30:306.

2. Meghan Butryn, Suzanne Phelan, James Hill, Rena Wing. Consistent self-monitoring of weight: a key component of successful weight loss maintenance. Obesity 2007;15:3091-96.

20: FACTS AND MYTHS

There will always be skeptics of any diet. However, if the concerns cannot be addressed with sound scientific principles, then the concerns should be dismissed as invalid. Conversely, the people who raise the question usually have no scientific evidence to back up their accusations. Rather, they often say, " I heard someone said…"

Opponents of our diet may raise the questions listed below. We are going to show you that there is no health risk or major side effects associated with this diet when it is followed correctly.

Does a high protein diet cause kidney or liver disease? There is plenty of research that shows this kind of diet is extremely safe for your kidneys and liver. The problem is when the patients already have *significant pre-existing* renal or hepatic disease; they cannot handle the protein load. Patients with pre-existing renal and/or hepatic disease should *not* be on this diet. A pre-diet and post-diet renal and liver function test will be ordered to show that this diet does not cause kidney or liver damage. People who worry that the high protein intake can cause renal damage should note that obesity is one of the main causes of end stage renal disease through the development of diabetes and hypertension.

There is not a single medical study to date that can link protein consumption to renal or liver damage in a patient with healthy kidney and liver function.

The Canadian Diabetic Association and the American Diabetic Association do not endorse the high-protein low-carbohydrate diet because they said that they do not have enough data to show that the diet is safe. However, they also do not have any data to show that the diet is not safe. They agree that this type of diet can help patients to lose weight and achieve better blood glucose control. However, they worry that the weight loss may not be permanent and this type of diet may elevate the bad cholesterol (LDL). Can they tell us which diet could provide permanent weight loss, even if the patient goes off the diet? If the patient stays with the diet plan, how can the patient re-accumulate fat? For patients who are on this diet, the LDL cholesterol usually ends up stable or improved. It is because this is not just a high-protein low-carbohydrate diet; it is also a low-in-animal-fat diet. There are studies that show that for normal patients and Type 2 diabetic patients, eating protein amounts twice the recommended daily allowance does not cause kidney damage; especially if the patients stay on a low salt diet and keep their blood pressure under good control[1].

Studies that demonstrated the negative effect of protein consumption on chronic renal failure were all done mostly with animal models. If this is true, then eating a diet that is low in protein should be able to halt the deterioration of the failing kidney. For people who have lost 50% of the GFR, the renal function will usually continue to deteriorate even when the cause of the failure has been removed. There have been so many patients on high protein diets over the last ten to twenty years, but there has yet to be case-reports linking protein consumption with kidney diseases. Maybe someone should look for kidney disease in carnivores. Since all they eat are protein and fat, all of their kidneys must be shot. Anssi H. Manninen in a review article concluded, "the American Heart Association Nutrition Committee's statement of dietary protein and weight reduction contains misleading and incorrect information. Certainly, such public warnings should be based on a thorough analysis of the scientific literature, not unsubstantiated fears and misrepresentations." For individuals with normal renal function, the risks are minimal and must be balanced against the real and established risk of continued obesity[2]. The opposite may in fact be true. Patient who followed a chicken based diet actually had improved the renal function and diminished microalbumin excretion[3]. In a study done on the pediatric population, research shows that there is no data indicating that a protein intake three to four times above the requirements has any adverse effects[4].

Creatinine Clearance (CC) is a commonly used laboratory test to assess renal function. It is an indirect measurement of the glomerular filtration rate (GFR). In general, the higher the GFR, the better the renal function. Protein intake appears to increase the renal blood flow and GFR[5]. On the other hand, protein-restricted diets have been shown to reduce renal blood flow and GFR in patients with renal disease.[6].

Another way to estimate the GFR (eGFR) is to use a mathematical model called the Modification of Diet in Renal Disease equation (MDRD). It estimates the GFR using age, sex, country of origin and serum creatinine. Hence, when the laboratory reports the patient's serum creatinine, it also provides the eGFR. eGFR does not take the patient's height and weight into consideration, whereas the Croft-Gault equation (CG) does. MDRD uses a standard surface area of 1.73 m[2]. Does this apply to all other ethnic groups? No - it does not apply to ethnic groups other than the African American and Caucasian populations.

MDRD formula:

GFR (mL/min/1.73m) = 186 x (creatinine)-1.154 x (age)-0.203 x (0.742 if female) x (1.210 if African American)

Cockcroft-Gault equation (CG):

GFR = (140-age) x weight in kg / serum creatinine in mmol/L

Although CG is by no means the standard method to estimate CC, it does take the patient's weight into consideration. CG can actually overestimate the CC of the obese patients because this group of patient is usually over weight in fat and water, rather than lean muscle mass. Underestimation of the CC using the eGFR method in this group of patient can produce unnecessary anxiety. With a low eGFR, physicians might hesitate to start or continue metformin. eGFR has limited usefulness in our obesity clinic. The old fashioned 24 hours CC test is still the method of choice in this group of patients[7].

The recommended daily allowance of protein is 0.8 g per kg of body weight. A study by Poortmans et al concluded that an athlete could safely ingest as much as 2.8 g per kilogram of body weight of protein each day[8]. This translates to 196 gram of protein per day for a 70 kilogram individual. Three oz of roasted skinless chicken breast contains 27 gram of protein. This is to say that you can eat 22 oz (1.4 pounds) of chicken breast per day without worrying about kidney damage.

Take, for example, two sets of renal patients: one follows a regular protein diet and the other follows a low protein diet. The GFR will be the same after 4 years on their respective diets if both groups are taking ACE inhibitor[9].

Patients with only a single solitary kidney will have a decreased that is usually stable, or slowly deteriorates. Increasing the GFR with protein is not beneficial because it put more pressure on the glomeruli and eventually leads to renal damage. However, if you induce post renal dilatation with an angiotensin converting enzyme inhibitor, increasing the GRF with protein consumption does not cause damage. Maybe it is due to the decrease in the pressure at the glomeruli.

Back in the 60's, the protein shake diet was very popular. People replaced *all* their meals with protein shakes. They did not eat anything else. Soon people died of heart attacks and it was the lack of mineral and vitamins in the protein shakes that posed the health problems, and not the excess of protein.

It was found that soy protein is less harmful to the damaged kidney than animal protein. Hence, soy protein shakes are allowed on the Phase 2 diet. Make sure that it does not contain an excessive amount of net carbohydrates.

Fluid is less satiating than solid foods[10]. Four hundred and fifty calories of sweetened fruit drinks produce a significant increase in body weight that was not found when the same amount of calories was consumed in solid form by the same individual.

Does your diet cause weight loss because you lose body water? It is true that there is a lot of free water loss during the first two weeks, but this will not be an ongoing phenomenon. This kind of water loss exists in all kinds of diet plans. The most convincing proof that you are actually losing fat is the presence of ketones in your urine and the loss of inches from your waistline. While plants store the extra sugar as starch, humans store sugar as glycogen. Glycogen is made from many sugar (glucose) molecules joined together by water to form a compact, highly branched, spherical structure. During the Induction Phase, glycogen from muscle (300 g) and liver (70 g) is metabolized and used up within the first three days. As the glycogen is broken down into smaller glucose molecules, water molecules associated with the glycogen molecule are released and eliminated via the kidney. You should see it as an advantage. An obese patient usually has water retention as shown by the presence of pitting edema in the limbs. Many obese patients are also hypertensive. They take diuretics just to get rid of the extra water via sodium loss by the kidneys. This diet promotes the elimination of free body water and improves peripheral edema and hypertension. If you start to consume excessive amounts of carbohydrates, the extra blood glucose will be stored as glycogen in the muscles and liver. Water will be retained by the glycogen molecule and cause a sudden increase in weight.

Water loss during dieting is due to:

1. Decreased insulin levels - decrease in insulin medicated renal tubular sodium reabsorption. Hence, decrease in extracellular and intravascular volume.

2. Utilization of glycogen, 3 to 4 g of water per g of glycogen.

3. Utilization of muscle, 19-25 g of water per g of nitrogen.

4. Utilization of fat, 10-15% of fat is water[11].

Your diet promotes ketogenesis. Is it harmful to your health? It is the intention of this diet to promote fat burning. It is perfectly safe. Please refer to Chapter 8.

This diet depletes stored glycogen. Does your diet decrease exercise tolerance and performance? The obese patient that needs to go on this diet is not going to perform in the Decathlon at the Olympics. Most of them do not do much exercise in the first place. By losing some weight on this diet, a patient will feel lighter and will be able to do more exercise than before. The body will be using fat as the main source of fuel while the patient is doing physical activities and this is the exact objective of this diet, to have the patient burn off the excess body fat.

Does your diet cause bad breath and constipation? If you follow the diet plan, you should not be constipated. However, your bowel habits may change from having a bowel movement daily to every second or third day in Phase 1. If you really suffer from hard bowel movements, then one should increase the fiber in their diet. Scandinavian Bran Crispbread®, Sugar-free Metamucil®, Metamucil® capsules, Prodiem® , and flaxseed are good choices. However, it will take 3 to 4 days before they start to work. Drink plenty of water with them. These fibers help to bind up cholesterol and bile in the intestine and excrete them out of the body. Hence, they can help to lower serum cholesterol. Fiber may also help to prevent colon cancer. Eating fiber decreases the chance of diabetes. Diabetes is infrequent in rural Africa, which may be the result of a high consumption of unprocessed carbohydrates. On Phase 2, you will be eating breads and cereals that are high in fiber but low in absorbable carbohydrates. The recommended Daily Allowance for fiber is 20 to 30 g. One serving of the Fibre 1® cereal gives you 16 g of fiber. Five Metamucil® capsules contain only 3 g of fiber. Vegetables and fruits that you are allowed to eat on this diet contain good amounts of fiber. Half a cup of cooked cabbage contains 1.7 g, broccoli contains 2.3 g, spinach contains 2.9 g, blueberries contain 2.0 g, and raspberries contain 4.2 g.

If you are having difficulty with bowel movements, you may take two Surfak capsules daily. If you need immediate results, you may take two tablets of Senokot® or a cup of Senna tea at bedtime and repeat as needed. Diet green tea usually has some laxative effects. Other than constipation, bad breath might result from the production of high amounts of ketones in the blood while you are burning fat (a good effect). Simply drink more water and this will flush out the blood ketones via the kidney. You may chew sugarless gum.

Dietary fibers come from the parts of plants resistant to digestion and absorption. It can be either soluble or insoluble. Insoluble fiber such as cellulose absorbs moisture and increases the fecal bulk, softens the stool and increases in transit time. Soluble fiber such as pectin helps with cholesterol reduction by binding bile acids and helps with metabolism of glucose and cholesterol synthesis by the way of intra-colonic fermentation. Soluble fiber produces short-chain fatty acids and gets absorbed via the portal circulation. Hence, soluble fibers do contain certain amounts of calories. By definition, any plant products that are not completely digested and are fermented by the colonic flora can be considered as "soluble fiber". Many sugar alcohols behave this way. Inulin, an extract from chicory root, has a sweet taste and low calorie content. It promotes the growth of normal colon flora and gets fermented into short-chain fatty acids. The sweetener that behaves like a fiber. Polydextrose, erythritol, maltitol, Xanthan gum and guar gum are all soluble fibers that are commonly used as thickening agents to thicken dishes.

Table 41. Nutritional Values of Some of the Commonly Used Grain Products.					
Flour Type (¼ cup)	Total Carb (g)	Fibre (g)	Net Carb (g)	Fat (g)	Protein (g)
White	23	1	22	0	3
Whole Wheat	22	3	19	1	5
Spelt	22	2	20	1	4
Soy	9	4	5	5	9
Rye (dark)	22	7	15	1	5
Rye (light)	20	4	16	1	2
Quinoa	24	5	19	2	4
Oat Bran	24	3	21	1	3
Kamut	25	2	21	0.5	4
Millet	16	2	24	1	4
Buck-wheat	28	2	26	1	5
Almond	4	3	1	12	5
Gluton	5	0	5	0	23
Flax Seed	13	11	2	14	6

Flax seeds and almonds contain very high amounts of fiber and low amounts of net carbohydrates. I have been asked by patients if they can eat bread products made with spelt flour. As you can see from table 41, spelt flour contains 20 grams of net-carbohydrates and only 2 grams of fiber. This is only marginally better than white flour. Hence you are not allowed to eat bread that is made from spelt flour in either Phase 1 or 2.

Is your diet nutritionally balanced? During the Induction Phase, you are not allowed to have dairy products and you may worry about the lack of calcium in this diet. However, calcium comes from many other sources, like broccoli. Cheese, nuts, and yogurt will be reintroduced to your diet slowly. Postmenopausal females and people with a lot of urine ketones will be given a calcium supplement. You will be getting the entire required daily vitamin and mineral allowance from eating protein, fat and vegetables only. People who are on low protein diets (vegetarian diet) often develop vitamin B deficiency. A fat free diet can cause fat-soluble vitamin deficiencies (vitamin A, D, E, and K). Although there are thousands of species of organic molecules in our bodies, we only require 23 essential organic compounds and water to stay healthy. We have to consume 9 essential amino acids, 2 essential fatty acids, 13 vitamins, and 15 elements from our food sources to stay healthy. Please note that carbohydrates are not considered as essential because their elimination from our diets does not produce illness[12].

Critics of this diet always say that one has to eat a "balanced diet". However, they also usually tell the patients that saturated fat is to be avoided. Should patients consume saturated fat in order to make it a "balanced diet"? Why did the critics tell the patients to avoid eating saturated fat? The answer will be because saturated fat is not good for the patient since it will increase the LDL cholesterol level. A diet that has very low amounts of saturated fat is still considered as balanced diet. If I said that consuming carbohydrates is bad for obese patients with diabetes, shouldn't this diet then be considered as balanced too.

Who define the "balance diet"? Does it mean to eat some of everything? Does it mean the Canadian Food Guide is the balance diet? If you avoid eating sugar, does it mean that it is not a healthy balance diet and be detrimental to your health? Should diabetic patients eat sugar to "balance' their diet? How can you tell an obese person to eat fat and starches to satisfy the guideline of the Canadian Food Guide?

Thirty years ago, the Canadian Food Guide included butter and other high fat dairy products as part of a balance diet. Today, the latest version of the Food Guide told us not to eat them. Using the standard that was set 30 years ago, today's Food Guide recommendation will not be considered as a "balance diet".

I consider the Canadian Food Guide as a balance diet for the normal and Dr. Poon's Metabolic Diet as a balance diet for the obese.

Does your diet cause gallstone formation and biliary colic? Any time that you alter the composition of your diet, not just with this low-fat low-carbohydrate diet, you are changing the composition of your bile. This may lead to the formation of gallstones. When you stop dieting, you also increase your chances of gallstone formation. Another mechanism proposed by scientists to explain the formation of gallstones is called *biliary stasis*. Biliary stasis means that the bile sits inside the gall bladder without movement starts to crystallize to form stones. This diet allows certain amounts of good fat. Once the food reaches the small bowel, the gallbladder will contract and empty the bile into the gut to help with fat digestion. Hence there is less chance of biliary stasis. For the high carbohydrate and low fat diet, the gallbladder will not empty its contents and there is more chance of causing biliary stasis. Gallstone disease is related to age, female gender, hormone replacement, contraceptives, pregnancy, obesity and rapid weight loss in obese patients.

Does this diet contain too much fat? We have shown you before that you need to replace the *essential fatty acids* daily to maintain good health. You cannot manufacture these essential fatty acids from any other food sources. Research has shown that if you are on a low carbohydrate diet, high fat consumption has no ill effect on your health especially when you consume "good" fat. This diet is actually able to decrease the triglycerides level in the blood. On the other hand, a high-carbohydrate-low-fat diet has been shown to increase the triglycerides level in the blood. This diet discourages the use of saturated fat and trans fat (found in some margarines, milk and deep fried foods). There are a lot of misconceptions about the association between meat, shellfish, and fat. It is the fatty part of the meat that contains cholesterol and saturated fatty acids. The lean part of the muscles that you are supposed to eat is mainly protein. The organ meats (liver, brain, or intestines) contain high cholesterol levels that are not allowed in our diet. The same thing is true regarding shellfish. Bad fat and cholesterol are present in the fatty parts and the internal organ of the shellfish. If you eat the muscle part, like the lobster tail or the muscle of the scallop, you are eating mainly protein. This is why this diet does not allow you to eat the whole lobster, the whole shrimp, the whole mussel, the whole clam, or the whole oyster. When you eat oysters, you are swallowing not just the muscle, but also the liver, intestine, and all the organs, which are high in fat and cholesterol.

Does your diet cause leg cramps? Because *ketones* act as a powerful diuretic, you may be losing more electrolytes than you anticipate. A simple blood test will find out if you are losing too much sodium and/or potassium etc. If needed, a supplement will be prescribed to you. Do not take prescription-strength potassium supplement without a physician's approval. High blood potassium can also be harmful to your health.

What happens to my potassium if I do not eat a banana or drink a glass of orange juice daily when I am taking water pills? It is written on the pill bottle that I should eat them daily! Yes, banana and orange juices do contain more potassium than some fruits and vegetables. However, as shown in the table 42, you can obtain your daily potassium requirement from many other food sources.

Table 42. Potassium Content (mg) in some Commonly Eaten Foods.

Food	Quantity	Potassium (mg)
Lettuce, iceberg, raw	1 cup	83
Nuts, almonds	10 nuts	100
Apple, with skin	1	147
Strawberries, raw	1 cup	253
Turkey, light meat	3 oz	256
Broccoli	1 cup	278
Celery, raw	1 cup	312
Fish, salmon, cooked	3 oz	318
Orange juice	1 cup	325
Steak, top sirloin	3 oz	342
Banana	1	422
Bok Choy, cooked	1 cup	630
Spinach, cooked	1 cup	838

Source: USDA National Nutrient Database for Standard Reference, Release 16-1

Do not drink juice. Fluid is less satiating than solid foods[13]. Four hundred and fifty calories of sweetened fruit drinks produced a significant increase in body weight that was not found when the same amount of calories was consumed in solid form by the same individual.

Does your diet allow the use of artificial sweeteners? There are many kinds of artificial sweeteners on the market that are readily available. The first one is saccharin. The FDA no longer claims that *saccharin* is a cancer-causing agent if taken in moderate amounts. One bad side effect of using saccharin is that it can stimulate the pancreas to release insulin. It also leaves a bitter after-taste. *Cyclamate (Sweet'N Low and Sugar Twin™)* is thirty times sweeter than sugar and is sold in Canada and the United Kingdom but is banned in the United States. There is no evidence that it causes cancer. It contains 0.5 g of carbohydrates per package. *Aspartame (Equal™)* is a sweetener that is two hundred times sweeter than sugar. It has 0.5 g of carbohydrates per teaspoon. Since it does not have a bitter after-taste like saccharin, it is used in diet pop extensively. However, it is not stable in heat and cannot be used in cooking. *Sucralose (Splenda™)* has been available in Canada for many years. It is six hundred times as sweeter than sugar. It also has no after-taste and it is stable in heat. It is going to replace aspartame in diet pop soon. Splenda is not carbohydrate free. It carries 0.5 g of carbohydrates per teaspoon and only 1/8th the calories of sugar. No ill effect has been reported to date. *Acesulfame Potassium (Sunett™)* is the newest sweetener and is about 200 times sweeter than sugar. *Stevia* is a natural sweetener extracted from a plant. It has no calories and has no side effects. Some preparations of Stevia may cause after-taste effects. It has been recently approved by the FDA to use in diet soft drinks.

There are other natural sweetener used in diet products like *Sorbitol, Mannitol, Maltitol, Lactitol, Isomalt, hydrogenated starch hydrolysate, Erythritol and Xylitol.* These are called *sugar alcohols.* Sometime sugar alcohols are listed as *polyols.* Sugar alcohols can be found naturally in plants, trees and fruits. Unlike glucose or sucrose, the aldehyde and ketone groups of these carbohydrate molecules are changed into a hydroxyl group (hydrogenated carbohydrates), which has a similar structure as alcohol; hence the term sugar alcohol. Just like artificial sweeteners, sugar alcohols do not trigger the release of insulin because it gets absorbed very slowly.

Unlike artificial sweeteners, *sugar alcohol has calories.* Hence artificial sweeteners are also called *non-nutritive sweetener,* and sugar alcohol is called *nutritive sweetener.* Another word that can be used to describe sugar alcohols is *partially absorbed sugar.* Only part of these sugar molecules gets absorbed into the body. Hence the caloric value of sugar alcohol is lower than that of glucose (Tables 43 and 44). However, if there is a lot of sugar alcohol in the gut, it can result in flatulence or diarrhea. The weight of the sugar alcohol will be listed on the food label as part of the total carbohydrate count. You have to subtract the weight of the sugar alcohol from the total carbohydrate content to arrive at the "Net Effective Carbohydrates" or "Net Carb".

If you consume a lot of sugar alcohol, the calories will add up and affect the total energy balance. Although sugar alcohol does not trigger an insulin response and does not cause a quick rise in the blood sugar, it can still cause *weight gain* or *trigger an insulin response if over-consumed.*

How much sugar alcohol should be present in a food product before it is considered to be unsafe to eat? As a general rule, this diet does not want you to eat any products that contain more than 5 g of carbohydrates per serving. It was found that if the product contains more than 5 g of carbohydrates per serving, it might trigger an insulin response. However, it still partially depends on the glycemic index of that particular carbohydrate. As for sugar alcohol, since it contains about half the calories as glucose, a rule of thumb is to limit the sugar alcohol to 10 g per serving to avoid raising the blood sugar level, assuming that you eat one serving at a time. Conversely, if the food product only contains 2 g of sugar alcohol and no other form of sugar, than it will be safe to consume 5 serving at a time without affecting the blood glucose.

Maltodextrin is a carbohydrate molecule formed from maltose molecules. It has similar properties as dextrose (glucose). It has a very high glycemic index of 100 and carries 4 calories per gram. It should be included in the net-carb count so does not count as sugar alcohol.

In general, the net-carb count of a food product will be the sum of the weight of sugar, starch and maltodextrin.

Another type of minimally absorbable sugar molecule frequently used in diet products is called *Polydextrose (Litesse®)*. The food industry uses Polydextrose as a bulking agent, thickening agent, as sugar or a fat substitute. It is a synthetic sugar molecule binding glucose (Dextrose) with 10% Sorbitol and 1% citric acid. The FDA approved it's use in 1981. Polydextrose is resistant to digestion in the small intestines. Hence it only carries 1 calorie per gram and has a very low glycemic index of 5. When Polydextrose reaches the large intestine, partial fermentation occurs and leads to physiological effects consistent with dietary fiber. The result will be reduced fecal transit time, softened stools and an increased in the growth of favorable microflora. Diarrhea is the main side effect. A laxative effect may occur with the ingestion of more than 30 g of sorbitol. Studies show that patients lose weight if they take Polydextrose daily. Polydextrose in the diet does not affect the absorption of other nutrients. The carbohydrate content of Polydextrose is part of the total carbohydrate count, but not part of the "Net Effective Carbohydrate" count. Another word that can be used to describe Polydextrose is *partially absorbed starch*.

Another partially absorbed starch that needs to be mentioned is Inulin. Inulin is an oligosaccharide (7 to 8 dextrose molecules linked together) that can be found in chicory root and many other plants. Even though it is sweet, the glycemic index is very low and has minimal effects on blood glucose and insulin levels. Inulin is part of the total carbohydrate count but not the net-carb count. This diet allows 30 g of Inulin or Polydextrose per serving. Food industries have been adding inulin to their food products and then count it as soluble fiber. They also use a term called preprobiotic to describe Inulin. It stimulates the growth of lactobacilli (probiotic). Partial enzymatic hydrolysis of inulin results in the production of oligofructose, which enhances satiety, improves glucose control in hyperglycemic subjects, raises levels of plasma glucagon-like peptide 1, and improves blood lipid profiles. Glucagon-like peptide 1 (GLP-1) is produced primarily by the intestines in response to caloric intake, mainly from carbohydrates and fat. It increases insulin concentration and increases insulin sensitivity.

Since there are so many types of sugar alcohols, if only one type is used in a food product, it will be labeled using the actual name of that sugar alcohol. If more than one type of sugar alcohol is used in the food product, it will be labeled simply as "sugar alcohol". Not all sugar alcohols have the same glycemic indexes or calories. Maltitol has the highest number of calories per gram (3) and the highest glycemic index (50). It can raise the blood sugar enough to trigger an insulin response. It is difficult to remember all the numbers. Hence, for simplicity, I set the maximum amount of sugar alcohol allowed per serving to 10 g (Table 24).

Table 43. Calories per gram of Different Food Groups.	
Polydextrose and Inulin	1.0 calorie per gram
Sugar alcohols	2.6 (average) calories per gram
Carbohydrate, (sugar, starch and maltodextrin)	4.1 calories per gram
Protein	5.3 calories per gram (effective calories is 4 calories per gram in human)
Alcohol	7.0 calories per gram
Fat	9.3 calories per gram

The FDA has recently announced that all approved sweeteners in the market are safe to use and has no evidence that they can cause cancer in humans.

If you are really into label reading, you may wish to learn about the properties of different sugar alcohols. They are not created equally. Remember that pure glucose provides 4 calories per gram. Table 44 lists the calories per gram for different types of sugar alcohols commonly found in diet products.

Table 44. Glycemic index and calories per gram of different sugar alcohols.		
Name of Sugar Alcohol	**Glycemic Index**	**Calories per Gram**
Glycerol (Glycerine)	?	4.0
Maltitol	40-50	3.0
Polyglycitol	39	3.0
Xylitol	13	3.0
Sobitol	9	2.5
Isomalt	9	2.0
Lactitol	6	2.0
Mannitol	0	1.5
Erythritol	0	0.2

Of all of the sugar alcohols, glycerol has the highest amount of calories per gram. It has the same amount of calories as glucose because glycerol can be turned into glucose through a process called gluconeogenesis in the liver. However, this is a very slow process. Hence when glycerol is ingested, it will be used up as energy rather than go through gluconeogenesis. So what is the advantage of using it as a diet product? There are two major reasons that glycerol is beneficial in helping with weight and diabetic control. It does not raise the blood glucose level and does not trigger an insulin response. One thing that is not known yet is the exact glycemic value of glycerol. However, since it does not increase the blood glucose level, its glycemic index was estimated to be low.

Table 43. Chemical Properties of Different Kinds of Sugar Alcohols.

Monosaccharide:	
Sorbitol	Hydrogenation of glucose
Mannitol	Isomer of Sorbitol
Xylitol	5 carbon, naturally occurring
Erythritol	4 carbon, naturally occurring
Disaccharides:	
Maltitol	Hydrogenation of maltose
Isomalt	naturally occurring
Lactitol	naturally occurring
Oligosaccharides:	
Inulin	Fructose polymer with a terminal glucose,
Hydrogenated starch	naturally present or synthetic
Hydrolysate (HSH or	Structure similar to sorbitol, maltitol or a combination
polyols)	of a few types of sugar alcohols.
Polysaccharides:	
Polydextrose	Dextrose 89%, sobitol 10%, citric acid 1%

Maltitol is not as good a product as other sugar alcohols. Its glycemic index is high at 40-50 (varies with products) and carries 3 calories per gram. Hence it will elevate the blood glucose and trigger insulin responses, but to a lesser extent than pure glucose. The best sugar alcohol will be Erythritol because it does not influence the blood sugar level and carries no calories. If you happen to find products that contain sugar alcohol, buy the one with Erythritol and avoid using Maltitol.

Have you ever considered eating "real sugar" or "natural sugar" as unhealthy? These sugars have been found to cause obesity and worsen diabetes. Obesity also causes cancer, heart disease, stroke and clots. How come no one voices their concern when they feed their children candies, ice cream, chocolate milk and juice boxes? The adverse effect of sugar has been proven. The reverse is true for sweeteners; the potential adverse effect has never been proven. What are we afraid of? The public is totally misinformed. Doctors practice evidence-based medicine. We rely on clinical studies to determine if a product is safe. Until there are further studies to show that consuming the same quantity of sweetener is unsafe, I will continue to support the use of sweeteners.

Do I need to eat carbohydrates for good health? Because your diet is low in fruits and grains, does your diet lack vitamins and phytochemicals? This is a low carbohydrate and not a no carbohydrate diet. Do not mistake "no starch" for "no carbohydrate". Since there is no bread, pasta and rice in the Phase 1 diet, it should be labeled as "no starch". However, patients are allowed to eat vegetables, and vegetables all contain carbohydrates (fiber and sugar); it cannot be labeled as "no carbohydrate". The daily allowance of 300 g of carbohydrates proposed by the Canada Food Guide is totally arbitrary. There is no scientific evidence that you need 300 g of carbohydrates to stay healthy. Look at the lions. They only eat protein and fat, and hardly any carbohydrates. Look at the sharks; they only eat fish and they seldom develop cancer. Our ancestors were carnivores and ate meat, or maybe some fruits. The Eskimo diet mainly consists of animal fat and meat, yet they live a healthy life just like everybody else. Their risk of developing metabolic syndrome was very low in the past when they have not had much carbohydrate intake. With modern transportation and the availability of carbohydrates, Eskimos, especially the female has become fatter and the rate of increase in people suffering from metabolic syndrome is on the rise. The rate of rise is much faster than the rest of the United States14. It is true that you need glucose for energy. However you do not need to eat carbohydrates at all to produce glucose. Your body can make glucose from protein and fat. On the other hand you cannot manufacture essential amino acids or essential fatty acids from glucose. If you want to take a multivitamin daily, you can. This diet can be minimal in calcium in Phases 1 and 2. Once the patient is in ketosis, we usually start them on calcium, magnesium and vitamin D or the Metabolic Diet Supplements. This diet allows you to eat a lot of green leafy vegetables, which have a low glycemic load. They contain most of the necessary vitamins and fiber. There is no need to eat fruits that contain much higher amounts of absorbable carbohydrates. Grain products contain a high amount of starch. They have been associated with some autoimmune diseases (Chapter 3). A patient showed Dr. Poon an article in spring 2004 from "Body, Mind & Spirit" quoting a registered dietitian and sports nutritionist in Toronto. She said, "Our bodies need carbohydrates. Glucose is the only fuel for the brain and if you don't have carbohydrates, you don't have glucose." This is not true. Our body does not need carbohydrate to make glucose. It is true that the brain uses mostly glucose as fuel, but our body can convert fat (only the glycerol portion of the triglycerides get transformed into glucose, the fatty acid part cannot be changed into glucose directly in mammals. It must be changed into ketones before we can utilize it as a source of energy) and proteins into glucose (gluconeogenesis) when the blood glucose is low. This is how our body can keep the blood sugar within a narrow range. When the blood glucose level is high, insulin will be secreted to remove the glucose from the blood and deposit it in the muscle, liver, or fat cells. When the blood glucose level is low, glucagon will take charge and increase the rate of conversion of glycogen, fat and protein into blood glucose. Glucose is the main energy source for the brain, but it is not the only source. The brain can also use ketones (coming from fatty acid metabolism) as an alternative energy source. This is one of the ways to prevent too much muscle wasting during starvation. Carnivores are by definition creatures that eat only meat. They do not eat carbohydrates. If what the dietician said is true, all carnivores should have brains that do not function properly.

You do not have to rely on fruit to provide you with dietary fiber. The Canada's Food Guide suggests that you should have at least 25 g of fiber intake per day. It can be easily achieved with this diet plan.

Table 46. Fiber Contents of Some of the Commonly Eaten Food in Phase 1 and 2 of the Dr. Poon's Metabolic Diet Plan.		
Food Item	**Serving Size**	**Fiber (g)**
Bowel Buddy Bran Wafer*	1 biscuit	4.0
Broccoli, cooked	1 cup	5.1
Cabbage, cooked	1 cup	2.9
Cauliflower, cooked	1 cup	3.3
Celery, raw	1 cup	1.9
Cucumber, raw with peel	1 cup	1.5
Hi-Lo cereal*	½ cup	7.0
Hummus*	2 tbsp	0.8
Kale, cooked	1 cup	2.6
Okra, cooked	1 cup	5.2
Green pepper, raw	1 cup	2.5
Scandinavian Bran Crispbread*	1 piece	5.0
Soybean nut*	¼ cup	5.0
Spinach, cooked	1 cup	4.3
SMAP cereal*	½ cup	7.0
Turnips, cooked	1 cup	3.1

*Items available at www.ontarionutrition.ca

Does eating a high protein diet cause your cholesterol level to rise? People equate eating meat with eating fat. The lean part of the meat itself is almost 100% protein. It is the fat that *attaches* to the meat that causes the cholesterol level to rise. I emphasize *lean meat* and avoiding animal fat. Trimming off the visible fat when you eat will eliminate most of the animal fat. Since you cannot separate the fat in regular ground beef from the meat part, it is not allowed in our diet unless it is extra-lean. Sources of fat should come from fish and olive oil. Do not confuse this diet with the Atkins diet, which allows salt and all kinds of animal fat, e.g. side bacon, whole egg, and cheese. High serum cholesterol is due to eating bad fat and carbohydrates and not from eating cholesterol.

Your diet promotes a lot of weight loss in the short term. Will I regain my weight once I go off the diet? This is the most common complaint when a patient comes into our office. "I lost 50 pounds on Weight Watchers™ (or Doctor Bernstein's Diet™, or Jenny Craig™, etc). However, I gained all my weight back, and more!" When you go into their diet history, you will find that the patient has returned to their old eating habits after stopping the diet program. The patient did not follow the maintenance program. The patient will regain the weight if he or she begins to eat the wrong way. It would be a surprise if the patient did not regain the weight. The diet did not fail the patient, but rather the patient failed the diet. Just like a home gym set up. It helps you to gain some muscle while you are doing the exercises. When you stop using the home gym, you lose the muscle that you gained. You cannot say that the home gym failed to work. You failed because you did not follow through with the plan. Just like using chlorine to control algae in the swimming pool. As long as you are using the chemical, there is no algae growth. When you stop using the chlorine, algae will start to grow. This does not mean that chlorine is ineffective towards algae control. You have to continue to use it to get the desirable effect. Obesity is a chronic disease that has no "cure," but it can be controlled. You need to be careful in choosing your food for the rest of your life. Lipoprotein lipase is an enzyme found in abundance near the fat cells in obese subjects, which facilitates the conversion of triglycerides in the circulation into fat storage inside the fat cells. The more lipoprotein lipase, the easier is to gain fat weight. It was found that even with major weight reduction, the lipoprotein lipase level did not return to normal. This may help to explain why obese people regain their weight and not because of the type of diet.

Does your diet require the use of diet pills? Diet pills do work as long as you take them. However, they can lead to dependence and addiction. Some of them do not even work. They should only be used under very special conditions. They are just an adjunct to a good diet plan. Ionamin®, Tenuate® and Meridia® are called anorexiants. They work by suppressing the appetite. This class of drug has many side effects (e.g. hypertension, headache, addiction, insomnia, palpitations, hives.) including some severe side effects (e.g. pulmonary hypertension). Hence, they should only be used in very special cases and for short periods only. Xenical® helps with weight loss by slowing down the absorption of fat from the gut. Some of the undigested fat will be excreted in the stool. If there is a lot of undigested fat in the stool, it can cause diarrhea. Last year, the Canadian government allowed the maker of Xenical® to market it as an adjunct therapy for overweight diabetic patients. Research showed that after a meal, the patients who took Xenical® had their blood glucose rise up more slowly than the patients who had a placebo. Hence, Xenical® may be able to minimize the hyper-secretion of insulin in this type of diabetic patients. As mentioned before, we eat fat along with carbohydrates to slow down the absorption of the carbohydrate (Chapter 9). Since Xenical® prevents the break down of fat in your meal, there is a consistently high level of fat in the intestine, which slows down the absorption of the carbohydrates and decreases the glycemic index of your meal. The amount of weight loss due to taking the diet pills alone is small as that compared with this diet. Studies found that after taking Xenical® or Meridia® for *one year*, the average weight loss was 5% to 10% of the original body weight. On this diet, patients are expected to lose 10% of their weight within *2 months*.

Experts say that drastic food-group-reduction is not good for your health. Is it true that this diet does not allow carbohydrates? Yes, this diet does not allow you to eat many carbohydrates in the first few weeks. Note that this is a *low* carbohydrate diet, not a *no* carbohydrate diet. In Phase 1, we are eating a lot of green leafy vegetables and which are carbohydrates. People correlate carbohydrates with bread, pasta or rice. They do not know that vegetables are mainly carbohydrates. There are only three main food groups. They are carbohydrates, protein and fat. Since vegetables are not protein or fat, they must be carbohydrates. More carbohydrate will be added back to your diet during Phase 2 and Phase 3. Not all carbohydrates are equal in nutritional values. This diet will not allow you to eat simple sugar but will allow you to eat the more complex carbohydrates. This diet tries to reduce but not eliminate all carbohydrates. All experts agree that no one should consume saturated fat. This does not mean that the experts are eliminating your fat intake; but to replace it with the better quality fat like the monounsaturated and polyunsaturated fats. There are differences between dieting to lose weight and dieting to maintain weight. You are restricted to low amounts of carbohydrates during the fat reduction phase, but you can have much more good quality carbohydrates when you are on Phase 3. Although there are thousands of species of organic molecules in our bodies, we only require 23 essential organic compounds and water to stay healthy. We have to consume 9 essential amino acids, 2 essential fatty acids, 13 vitamins, and 15 minerals from our food sources to stay healthy. Please note that carbohydrates are not considered as essential because eliminating them from our diet does not cause illness[15.]

Your diet does not let me eat cheese; will I develop osteoporosis? Eating protein and fat has no effect on bone mass. Inadequate protein intake compromises bone health and contributes to osteoporosis in the elderly[16]. If you are drinking more than 3 cups of caffeinated drinks per day while not taking calcium will lead to bone loss. An increase in dietary sodium will lead to an increase in sodium loss in urine. Urine calcium loss will also go up. Hence a low sodium diet will be more suitable for patients with osteoporosis.

In order to achieve your daily calcium requirement of 1500 mg, you will have to eat 50 oz (3 pounds) of 17% cheddar cheese, which gives you half a pound of fat and 5,000 mg of sodium. Almost all food products contain some calcium. Some countries have a very low consumption of diary products e.g. China, because of lactose intolerance. However, the incidence of osteoporosis is not any higher than that of North

America. If in doubt, take a supplement. In the animal kingdom, which adult animals drink milk? Which animals develop osteoporosis? What did the cow eat to provide you with the calcium in her milk? If you are suppose to drink milk as part of good health, how come the females of our species are unable to provide milk year round for all their off springs?

The human body is an amusing and complex machine. It can channel food energy to the part of the body that needs it the most. If you wish to build up your biceps, you have to put stress on those muscles such as by doing weight lifting. Healthy amount of good quality of protein intake daily is also necessary. Once you built your biceps and decided not to exercise anymore, your muscle bulk will slowly return to the original size.

Table 47. Calcium Content (mg) of Some Commonly Eaten Foods.		
Food Item	Serving Size	Calcium (mg)
Yogurt, low fat	8 oz	415
Milk, skim	1 cup	306
Cheese, cottage 1%	1 cup	138
Cheese, cheddar	1 oz	28
Soy milk, calcium fortified	1 cup	245
Cucumber, with skin	1 large	301
Spinach	1 cup	291
Tofu	½ block	190
Tomato	1 cup	180
Strawberries	1 cup	166
Fish, Halibut	½ fillet	159

"If you don't use it, you will lose it."

The same principle is true regarding to the bones. For the mammals that walk all day long, their bodies will make sure that their bones are strong so that they can hold up their bodies. Human is different. We have all kind of modern conveniences and we hardly need to walk. We have no time to exercise. There is no need to go to grocery store too often because we can buy in bulk and store them in our refrigerators. We can even order the grocery on-line and they deliver them right to your door. I remembered that my grandmother used to walk to the markets twice a day to buy fresh produces and meats. Automobiles, remote controls, computers etc have been changing our lifestyles and we become couch potatoes. Putting the physiological reasons and side effects of medications aside, as we grow older, fatter and do less exercise, our bodies sense that there are no need to maintain strong bones since we are no using them. The bodies will channel the energy away from bones and the bones will become osteoporotic. Astronauts are health people with health bones before they go to the outer space. As they stayed in the space station for a prolonged period of time, they all develop osteoporosis. It is because in the weightlessness condition in the outer space, the body senses that there is no need to maintain strong bones to carry the body around. I believe that the lack of activities is one of the main causes of osteoporosis and not dietary related.

Studies have shown the obese person has less chance to develop osteoporosis than non-obese counter part. It is likely because the obese patients put more stress on their bones as they ambulate. Their body will respond by making stronger bones. It was found that only weight bearing exercises increase bone mass. Swimming, for example, does not have the same effect as walking since swimming is not a weight bearing exercise.

Your diet allows half a grapefruit per day. However, the label on my pill bottle stated that I should not drink grapefruit juice while taking the medication; can I have grapefruit? The effect of grapefruit juice on the metabolism of medications was first discovered while testing a blood pressure pill called felodepine. When patients take felodepine with a glass of grapefruit juice, it produces a much more potent blood pressure lowering effect than with water. This effect only occurs when the patient takes felodepine in the oral form. When felodepine is given through the intravenous route, ingestion of grapefruit juice has no effect on the pharmacokinetics of the drug. Later, it was found that grapefruit juice enhances the absorption of felodepine in the small intestine. Under normal circumstances, only 15% of the oral dosage of felodepine passes through the bowel into the blood stream. Up to 85% of the drug gets destroyed by an enzyme system (cytochrome P450) present in the lining of the bowels. Grapefruit juice inhibits this cytochrome P450 system, which leads to an increase in the bioavailability of the drug. More felodepine gets through the bowel wall without being destroyed. This is why when the drug is given intravenously, grapefruit juice cannot enhance the availability of the drug since most of the drug is already present in the blood stream. Hence any medication (e.g. some antibiotics, antihypertensive medications and cholesterol lowering medications) that usually gets partially destroyed by this cytochrome P450 system when taken in the oral form can be affected by grapefruit juice. However, if you eat grapefruit in the morning and take your cholesterol pill in the evening, the absorption of the drug will not be affected. Some doctors suggested that it make more economical sense to take these drugs with grapefruit juice because you can achieve more bang for your buck. Taking 10 mg of Lipitor with grapefruit juice produces the same cholesterol lowering effect as 20 mg of Lipitor taken with water. However, the higher dosage of certain medications might produce side effects.

References:

1. Knight et al. The Impact of Protein Intake on Renal Function Decline in Women with Normal Renal Function or Mild Renal Insufficiency. Annals Internal Medicine 18 March 2003;138:460-467.

2. Anssi H. Manninen. High-protein weight loss diets and purposed adverse effects: where is the evidence? Sports Nutrition Review Journal 2004;I:4-51.

3. Jorge L. Gross et al. Effect of a chicken-based diet on renal function and lipid profile in patients with Type 2 diabetes. Diabetes Care 2002; 25:645-651.

4. Kim Fleischer Michaelsen. Are there negative effects of an excessive protein intake? Pediatrics Nov 2000;106 No. 5 supplement:1293.

5. Smoyer WE, Brouhard BH, Rassin DK et al. J Lab Clin Med 1991;118:166-75.

6. Hirschbery R, Kopple JD, Kidney Int 1987;32:382-7.

7. Poon P, Poon D, Wong M, Underestimation of Creatinine Clearance using the eGFR versus the Cockcroft-Gault Formula in the Obese Type 2 Diabetics Taking Insulin. Obesity Oct 2008;16 supplement 1:S113.

8. Poortman JR, Dellalieux O. Do regular high protein diets have potential health risks on kidney function in athletes? Int J Sport Nutr March 2000;10(1):28-38.

9. Hansen HP, Tauber-Lassen E, Jensen BR, et al. Kidney Int 2002;6:220-8.

10. DeMeglio and Mattes, Physiol Behav 1996;59:179-87.

11. Rudman D, Bleier J, Nutritional Requirements. Harrison's Principles of Internal Medicine. 10th edition. McGraw-Hull book company 1983. Page 426.

12. Nilsson LH. Scand J Clin Lab Invest 1973;32:317-23.

13. DeMeglio and Mattes, Physiol Behav 1996;59:179-87.

14. Naylor JL, Schraer CD, et al. Diabetes among Alaska Natives: a review. Int. J Circumpolar Health 2003;62:363-87.

15. Rudman D, Bleier J, Nutritional Requirements. Harrison's Principles of Internal Medicine 10th edition. McGraw-Hill Book Company 1983. Page 426.

16. Johnson LK, Lykken GI, et al. J Nutr 2003;133:1020-6.

"Carbohydrate is not considered as an essential nutrient because its deletion from the diet does not produce illness."

21: "I am a Stress Eater"

Patients often tell me that they are stress eaters or emotional eaters. That is the reason they became obese. What does "stress eater" or "emotional eater" mean?

The emotional eater eats when he or she becomes emotional. "I am sad, therefore I eat." Somehow the patient does not go for the healthy food; the patient usually went for the "comfort food" to feel better. There is no definition of "comfort food". It usually means high calorie, high sugar, high fat and/or salty foods. However, junk food usually does not provide comfort to the patient in the long run. When the patient starts to gain weight after eating the wrong type of food, further deterioration of health will follow. Instead of providing "comfort" to the patient, it provides the patient with "sadness".

The other side of sadness is happiness. Happiness is a kind of emotion also. "I ate a piece of cake because it was my son's birthday." Is there any law to say that I have to eat a piece of cake on my birthday? People tell me that it will just be once in awhile that they eat cake, such as at birthday parties. If they have big families, there will be many birthday parties. How about wedding parties, graduation parties, retirement parties, going away parties or the Stanley Cup party? If you wish to eat cake, you can always find an excuse. Eating cake on birthdays is a tradition and not because it is governed by religious rules or medical reasons.

Patients often ask me if it is ok if they "only eat sweets occasionally". I answer the question with a question of my own. I will ask the patient; if your children came up to you and asked for permission to snore cocaine, what would be your response? The answer will be a definite "no". If they modify their request and seek permission to snort cocaine "only occasional", your answer will still be "no". If they seek permission to snort cocaine once a year only on their birthday, will you agree?

Let's say that you have never cheated in an exam before; and the first time you cheated, you got caught by the teacher. It doesn't matter if you have a clean history; you are still guilty as charged.

Emotional eaters, eat when they are sad and they eat when they are happy. When will they stop? Do they have to be emotionless before they stop to eat? Do all normal weight people have no emotions?

Given the same situation, some people adapt beautifully and some people can become a total wreck. It depends on your personality. Is the cup half full or half empty? Why can't you be an optimist rather than a pessimist? Why can't you find the silver lining in every problem you have to face?

Let's say you got caught speeding. How are you going to react? You can start to cry and beg for forgiveness. You can start cursing and yell at the police. You can apologize to the police officer and take the ticket gracefully. You can fight the ticket in court. You can pay someone to fight for you in court. You can lose sleep over it. If that had been me, I would just take the ticket and pay someone to fight the ticket for me in court so that I would not have to lose points. I would consider myself lucky since I did not get into a serious accident even though I was speeding. I still arrived home safely. Whatever done is done; I cannot help it. No matter what, stress or no stress, it did happen. Not much I can do about it. I have to look ahead instead of asking myself "what if". This is part of life. There is nothing that I can do about things that

I have no control over, such as getting caught speeding. It happened already. If there is something that you can do, such as fight the ticket, then do it. Yes, I have to waste some money and time. At least I can do something about it. If I just get angry and start to "stress eat", the fact that I got caught still remains and the problem will not disappear by itself. No matter how much you stress, the problem will never go away on its own.

In medical school, a professor in psychiatry taught me that if ninety nine percent of the population reacts the same way that you react to a certain situation, then your reaction would be considered as normal. For example, most people will grieve the passing of their loved one for about six months. After six months of grieving, they started to live a life similar to that before the passing of their loved one. If you are still grieving for more than three years, your grieving has become pathological. Remember, life goes on with or without you.

You are reading this book, or coming to see me, in search of a diet to lose weight and regain your health. Good for you. For whatever reason, you need to give yourself incentive to go on a diet. If you tell me that "I am stressed, hence I cannot diet". I will tell you to forget about dieting. You will fail all diets. You are using "stress" as a trump card to give yourself a reason to cheat.

Everyone can give me a reason or reasons to deviate from the diet. However, there is never a good enough reason; a bank robber has a reason to rob the bank; a student has a reason to cheat in an exam; a murder has a reason to kill someone. Can the reasons justify their actions? I would also like to be a millionaire, but I cannot just go to rob a bank. I know the consequences for robbing the bank, so instead, I have to work harder so that maybe one day I become a millionaire. Dieting is the same thing. If you want to lose weight and regain your health you have to work hard for it. The consequence of stress eating is weight gain and death. I understand that everyone dies one day, but you do not have to die prematurely.

I hear from patients all the time that they are trying their best. They end up gaining weight. What do you mean when you are trying very hard? If your son, who you know is very smart, came home with all F's in his report card and he told you that he is trying very hard to get all A's, what are you going to say to him? You will likely say to him that he is NOT trying hard enough.

Everything is hard in life. It depends on how you let the situation run your life. Getting up on a cold winter morning to go to work is hard. Nevertheless, when I think of all the patients that I am helping, and that I may become a millionaire in the future, getting up in the morning is not so bad.

Everything in life is stressful. "My 98 year old aunt is sick, I am stressed." "The country is going into recession, I am stressed." "There is tension in the Middle East, I am stressed." The question is, what can you do about it? If you cannot do anything about it, it should not stress you out. You have to accept that this is part of life. Your aunt is supposed to get old, sick and eventually die. This happens to everyone, including you. No matter how you react to this situation, you are not going to change the inevitable. Learn from the optimist. The optimist will say that your 98 year old aunt is going to a better place with no more suffering and is going to meet all her friends and relatives who died before her.

These are things that you have no control over. There are going to happen with or without your input. However, you have complete control of the type of food that you put into your month. No one can force you to eat my birthday cake if you do not want to. If you are allergic to shellfish, you are not going to eat the shrimp dish that I told you that I had made especially for you, because you know that the consequence of eating the shrimp means death.

It sounds like that I am insensitive to people with psychological issues when I tell the patient not to start the diet because I do not think that the patient is ready. The patient should seek help from a psychologist instead. Going through with a diet requires the total commitment of the patient. The patient has to be mentally ready to change their eating habits, learn to cope with stress, start exercise, etc. If you are not ready, do not start any diet program. It will only lead to failure and you will feel more depressed. Honesty is the best policy. The truth can be difficult to accept.

If the patient did well losing weight, I would tell the patient that he/she is doing a good job. If the patient gains weight, I have no problem in telling the patient that he/she has been cheating, either knowingly or unknowingly. It is totally acceptable to admit to cheating and then to put more effort in following the program in the future. However, being defensive and lying will only be hurting oneself. The doctors at the clinic are there to guide the patients through the different phases of the diet plan and us the appointments as opportunity to teach patients about nutrition, facts and myths on dieting, and monitor their health status so that no harm will be done to the patients. Cherish it. Remember, the doctor can only help those who help themselves.

No one can make you eat it but yourself

22: Invasive and Non-invasive Bariatric Procedures

In 2006-7, there were a total of 100000 cases of bariatric surgery performed in the USA. Roux-En-Y gastric bypass was the most commonly done bariatric surgery. Fifty nine percent were laparoscopic gastroenterostomies (RYGB), Banding 12%, and gastrojejunostomy 29%[1].

Bariatric surgery is indicated for a patient who has a BMI of over 40. This is considered as the last option when conventional methods of weight control have failed[1]. The most beneficial effect of bariatric surgery is better glycemic control in the diabetic patient, after a substantial amount of weight loss.

There are pros and cons for different types of bariatric surgery. Prospective patients should receive full counseling about the facts of bariatric surgery, including side effects during and after surgery. The patient has to accept that there will have to be a big lifestyle change after the surgery. Patient selection is important to ensure that the surgical procedure will be successful. Bariatric surgery is contraindicated in patients with eating disorders and psychiatric conditions. Patients are encouraged to lose weight prior to surgery.

Table 48. Pros and Cons for Different Types of Bariatric Surgery.

Surgical Type	Pro	Con
Gastric Banding	No malabsorption, No dumping syndrome, Reversible, Can be use as a bridge until the patient can do other surgical procedure, Minimum surgical risk.	Needs adjustment, Does not decrease, Ghrelin production, Only moderate weight reduction, Slippage, Erosion.
RYGB	Large amount of weight reduction, Improve glycemic control, Less chance to regain.	Dehydration, vomiting, Dumping syndrome, Malabsorption, Anemia, Protein and vitamin deficiency, Obstruction, Depression, High mortality (1-2%), High morbidity (20%), Not reversible.
Intragastric Balloon	Non-invasive, Reversible, Can be removed easily, Well tolerated, Adjustable.	Good for 6 months only, Vomiting and reflux, Erosion, Obstruction, Migration, Not as effect as other 2 methods in weight reduction.

Because of their obesity, there is a higher risk of blood clot formation. Hence, the early complications are pulmonary embolism, hemorrhage, leak, wound infection, obstruction and atelectasis. Later, complications might include stoma sternosis, anastomotic leak/ulcer, hernia, nutritional deficiency, and dumping syndrome. Long term complications include outlet sternosis, band erosion, bowel obstruction, depression, incisional hernias, gall stones, and gastroesophageal reflux. There is a very high risk of developing depression post-operatively. Suicidal rate is high.

Dumping syndrome is common in patients post-gastric bypass surgery. It results from rapid emptying of stomach contents into the small bowel. There is malabsorption of carbohydrates and fat, which when passing into the large intestine, causes diarrhea. In order to minimize the symptoms of dumping syndrome, the patient should be following a diet that is small in quantity, low fat and low carb. This is very similar to the type of diet that Dr. Poon teaches. You can do Dr. Poon's diet without surgery or do the surgery and follow Dr. Poon's diet post-operatively.

Post gastric bypass surgery patients need to monitor their serum electrolytes, liver and renal functions, vitamin B12, protein, calcium, magnesium, and iron. For anemia, take two 300 mg iron sulfate tablets per day (for female patients, as long as you continue to menstruate). Patients may require B12 injections. B12 absorption is not complete with food. Watch out for thiamine deficiency, which can cause double vision, Wernicke's syndrome, ataxia, and beriberi. It can be treated with intramuscular thiamine injections. Calcium citrate is better than carbonate since these patients have a higher pH in the GI tract and the absorption of calcium citrate is more complete. Calcium citrate does not produce an elevated oxalate level, which can cause renal stones. Watch your Coumadin® and lithium levels post-op. The lithium level is affected by dehydration and sodium levels. Most patients have difficulty with eating vegetables and need to monitor their INR and may require less Coumadin®.

The intragastric balloon (Heliosphere®) procedure involves filling a balloon device within the stomach. The volume occupied promotes a sensation of satiety and weight loss. After inflating the balloon, the balloon acts as an artificial bezoar and moves freely in the stomach.

Reference:

1. National Institutes of Health. Clinical Guidelines on the Identification, Evaluation, and Treatment of Overweight and Obesity in Adults - the Evidence Report. Obes Res 1998;6(supp):51S-209S.

23: PHILOSOPHY OF DR. POON'S DIET

- If in doubt, don't eat it

- Learn to say "No, thank you"

- Money cannot buy you health

- Less Salt, Less Fat, Less Carb

- Never give up, do Phase 1 again

- A little bit of cheating is NOT OK

- Disease and diet do not take holidays

- Don't expect me to (S)Poon feed you

- Yo-yo dieting is worse than no dieting

- You will not die if you skip the dessert

- Diet does not fail you; you fail the diet

- No one can make you eat it but yourself

- Other people have done it, why can't you

- No adult animal except humans drink milk

- It is not how much you eat, but what you eat

- What kind of carbohydrate does the Eskimo eat

- Any amount of exercise is better than no exercise

- I would rather waste my money than waste my health

- Nobody can help you if you do not help yourself first

- Don't just say I want to lose weight, you have to DO it

- Treatment of a "stress eater" is to live a stress-free live

- Any amount of weight loss is better than no weight loss

- If you lose, you cannot gain. If you can't lose, don't gain

- When you lose, you lose muscle; when you gain, you gain fat

- Medication only treats a number, weight reduction treat the cause

- No such thing as finishing a diet, it is a permanent lifestyle change

- Everybody cheats, but some learn to get back on track the next day

- "Healthy eating" has nothing to do with weight loss or diabetic control

- Everyone has an opinion on diet, listen to the one with the diploma

- If you find a diet that works, is easy to follow and maintain, keep that diet

- Cow eat grass; they don't drink milk to provide you with calcium rich milk

- Fad diets are defined as any diet that you cannot sustain for the rest of your life

- Junk food is defined as any food that causes you to gain weight, raise your blood sugar or blood pressure

- "Natural" disaster is not better than man-made disaster, and "Natural" sugar is not better than refined sugar

24: Summary

I hope that you enjoyed reading this book. It is my intention to show you why I say eating too many carbohydrates, saturated fat and sodium can be bad for your health. Once you understand the principle behind Dr. Poon's Low-Carbohydrate-Low-Sodium-Low-Fat Diet, you will not be afraid to eat protein and good fat. I am looking not just weight loss, but also, for you to lose your body fat, quickly and safely. If you follow the plan, it is completely safe and you can do this for the rest of your life.

You are now slimmer, trimmer, and full of energy. You will be taking fewer medications than when you started the diet. Don't be afraid to tell your friends that you are on the diet. Spread the good news. I am sure more and more research is going to come out to substantiate my claim.

As a physician, I was able to see first hand how this diet improves the quality of life in obese patients. Many patients worry that once they are on anti-diabetic, anti-lipid, or antihypertensive medications, they will have to take them for life. I told them "not so". If they can change their eating habits and lifestyles, and are able to lose some fat and weight, then their disease will improve and I can safely eliminate or decrease some of their medications. For patients with metabolic syndrome, medication only treats the symptom and weight loss treats the cause. The fat that you accumulated in your belly all these years is the root of all evil. You should use medications to prevent disease and not rely on them to treat your obesity related diseases.

Newer technology has allowed us to process our food sources in an effective manner. However, all these refined sugars, flours and foods have given us modern day diseases like diabetes, coronary heart disease, indigestion and cancer.

Continue to exercise after the weight is lost. It is critical for weight maintenance.

For those who wish to help themselves, I am here to guide you through the different stages of this diet so that you will feel good and full of confidence once again.

If there is a diet that is easy to do and effective, do it. There is no end to any diet program. It is a lifestyle change. You will have to keep the diet for life. Do not give yourself any reason to go off the diet. You have to sacrifice something to gain something. In this case, you are sacrificing junk food to regain your health. Ultimately, you have to take responsibility for your own actions. Do not complain when you did not lose weight if you cheated on the diet. Accept the fact that you have made a mistake and return to the diet plan immediately. Do not have to give up dieting all together. Learn from your past mistakes.

It is not my intention to compete with the commercial programs. We do not see obese patients that are obese but are not suffering from obesity related diseases. Those patients can follow any commercial program such as the Weight Watchers™ diet and will be fine. However, if the patient has a complicated medical history, a physician should monitor the patient closely.

I am a clinician and not a researcher. I have no statistics to show you the rate of success of this diet. However, I can tell you this: You will lose weight, decrease your water retention, get your blood glucose under better control, improve on your lipid profiles and lower your blood pressure if you follow the diet diligently. I am doing a study to find out what percentage of patients who achieved their weight goal and maintained their weight for 1 to 2 years. Initial result was very encouraging. As far as I know, there is no medical textbook on the market that teaches doctors how to counsel their patients with metabolic syndrome to lose weight. This low-carbohydrate low-sodium low-fat diet plan is written in such a way that both the patients and the doctors can benefit from reading it. I am happy that there are many family physicians out there wanting to know more about this diet program, especially when they saw the benefits of this diet first hand in their patients. I hope that more physicians and dietitians will adopt the general principles of this diet in helping their patients to achieve their healthy weights. That will be the ultimate goal for me.

If you find a diet that works,
is easy to follow and maintain, keep that diet

25: About the Author

Dr. Poon moved from Hong Kong to the U.S. in 1975. He attended the University of Southern Mississippi and earned his Bachelor of Science Degree with Highest Honors in the Department of Medical Technology in 1978. Clinical Biochemistry was his area of interest. After working briefly at a local clinical laboratory, he decided to pursue further studies in Clinical Biochemistry. In 1979, he started his graduate studies in the Department of Pathology at the Medical College of Wisconsin in Milwaukee. Under the guidance of Professor Doumas, who is an authority in the analysis of serum protein and bilirubin, he received his Doctoral of Philosophy in 1983. During his graduate studies, he continued to work in the hospital, as well as research laboratories. The knowledge he accumulated from his laboratory experience and graduate studies provided him with the biochemistry background that was needed in designing this diet program later on.

After he immigrated to Canada, he studied medicine at the University of Toronto. He started his family practice career in Richmond Hill, Ontario since graduation in 1987. His interest in weight control began twenty years ago. However, his "low-fat and eat-less" Canada's Food

Guide approach did not have much success. One of his patients asked him for his opinion about a "high-protein diet", he began to study the mechanism of the "low-carbohydrate high-protein diet" and found that this type of diet did merit a clinical trial. In addition to low-carbohydrate, he designed a diet plan that is also low in saturated fat and low sodium. He found success in helping his patients to lose weight and improve on their health. Since that time there has been more formal research done on low-carbohydrate-high-fat diets. However, there is not much work done on low-carbohydrate low-fat diets yet. Dr. Poon has seen first hand the positive effect of his diet on his obese patients, especially those patients suffering from metabolic syndrome and Type 2 diabetes. The most gratifying moment is when he sees the happy faces of his diabetic patients when they go off insulin injections once they lose weight and get their blood glucose under good control. He has been an advocate of the low-carbohydrate low-fat low-sodium high-fiber diet ever since.

Dr. Poon's idea of a good diet program is not just to provide a diet plan for the patients, but also to educate them about the facts of nutrition and exercise. There are too many misconceptions out there. He believes that when the patients understand what to look for in a food product, they will be able to make better choices. Dr. Poon practice what he preaches and keeps his weight down. His cookbook contains recipes that his wife prepares for him that are low in fat, carbohydrates and salt. Exercise is encouraged. He calls his diet the "Healthy Diet for the Obese".

Being a Diplomat of the American Board of Physician Nutrition Specialist, Doctor Poon offers nutrition counseling to patients coming from all over North America. He appears in radio and TV shows, writes columns for newspapers and magazines, gives public speeches, and educates the medical communities.

Dr. Poon lives in Toronto, with his wife Beckie, his son Douglas and his daughter Rebecca.

Appendix

Food	Glycemic Index	Net-Carb (g per serving)	Glycemic Load
Fruits			
Apple, 1 medium	38	18	6.8
Apple, dried, 1 oz	29	24	7.0
Apricots, fresh, 3	57	12	6.8
Apricots, dried, 1 oz	29	24	7.0
Banana, 1	55	32	17.6
Blackberries, ½ cup	*46*	*5*	*2.3*
Blueberries, ½ cup	*50*	*8*	*4.0*
Cantaloupe, ½ cup	*65*	*4*	*2.6*
Cherries, 10	*22*	*10*	*2.2*
Dates, dried, 5	103	27	27.8
Durian, ½ cup		28	
Figs, dried, 2	75	20	15.0
Grapefruit, ½	*25*	*5*	*1.3*
Grapes, 1 cup	46	15	6.9
Guava, 1		*6*	
Honey dew, ½ cup	*68*	*5*	*3.4*
Jackfruit, 1 oz		*6*	
Juice, apple, ½ cup	59	14	8.3
Juice, cranberry, ½ cup	48	18	8.6
Juice, cherry, ½ cup	55	16	8.8
Juice, grape, ½ cup	69	19	13.1
Juice, grapefruit, ½ cup	48	11	5.3
Juice, guava, ½ cup		13	
Juice, lemon, 1 tbs		*1*	
Juice, lime, 1 tbs		*1*	
Juice, orange, ½ cup	46	13	6.0
Juice, tomato, ½ cup	*38*	*5*	*1.9*
Kiwi, 1	*52*	*8*	*4.2*
Lychee, fresh, 10		15	
Mango, 1	55	19	10.5
Nectarine, 1		14	
Orange, ½	*44*	*5*	*2.2*
Papaya, ½ medium	58	14	8.1
Passion fruit, 1		*3*	
Peach, fresh, 1 medium	*42*	*7*	*2.9*
Pear, 1	38	21	8.0

Food	Glycemic Index	Net-Carb (g per serving)	Glycemic Load
Fruits (continue...)			
Persimmon, 1		21	
Pineapple, 2 slices	66	10	6.6
Plum, 1	*39*	*7*	*2.7*
Pomergranate, 1		25	
Prunes, ½ cup	29	46	13.3
Raisins, ¼ cup	64	28	17.9
Raspberries, ½ cup	*44*	*3*	*1.3*
Strawberries, ½ cup	*40*	*4*	*1.6*
Watermelon, ½ cup	*72*	*4*	*2.9*
Nuts and Seeds			
Almond, 2 tbs		*1*	
Cashew, 25 g	*22*	*5*	*1.1*
Chestnuts, 6		24	
Flax seed, 3 tbsp		*5*	
Ginkgo nut, 1 oz		*10*	
Hazelnuts, 2 tbs		*2*	
Macadamia, 2 tbs		*1*	
Peanuts, 2 tbs	*21*	*2*	
Pecans, 2 tbs		*1*	
Pine nuts, 2 tbs		*2*	
Pistachio, 2 tbs		*3*	
Pumpkin seeds, 2 tbs		*3*	
Sesame seeds, 1 tbsp		*1*	
Soy nuts, 1/3 cup		*8*	
Sunflower seeds, 2 tbs		*2*	
Walnuts, 2 tbs		*1*	
Pastas			
Fettuccini, 1 cup	32	57	18.2
Gnocchi, 1 cup	68	71	48.3
Linguine, 1 cup	50	56	28.0
Macaroni, 1 cup	45	52	23.4
Ravioli, meat-filled, 1 cup	39	32	12.5
Spaghetti, white, 1 cup	41	52	21.3
Spaghetti, whole wheat, 1 cup	37	48	17.8
Tortelini, cheese, 8 oz	50	26	13.0
Vermicelli, 1 cup	35	42	14.7

Food	Glycemic Index	Net-Carb (g per serving)	Glycemic Load
Vegetables			
Avocado		15	
Artichoke, 1	*20*	*7*	*1.4*
Artichoke heart, 1	*20*	*1*	*0.2*
Asparagus spears, 6	*20*	*2*	*0.4*
Baked beans, ½ cup	48	24	11.5
Bamboo shoots, fresh ½ cup		*3*	
Barley, ½ cup	25	22	5.5
Bean sprouts, 1 cup		*4*	
Beet, raw 3 oz		*6*	
Black beans, ¾ cup	30	31	9.3
Black-eyed beans, ½ cup	42	16	6.7
Bok Choi, 1 cup	*20*	*1*	*0.2*
Broccoli, ½ cup	*20*	*2*	*0.4*
Brussels sprouts, 6	*20*	*8*	*1.6*
Cabbage, ½ cup	*20*	*1*	*0.2*
Cabbage, mustard, 1 cup		*2*	
Carrots, ½ cup	*60*	*5*	*3.0*
Carrot juice, 8 oz		26	
Cauliflower, 5	*20*	*2*	*0.4*
Celery stalk, 1	*20*	*1*	*0.2*
Celery root, ½ cup		*6*	
Chickpeas, canned, ½ cup	42	15	6.3
Corn, ½ cup	55	16	8.8
Couscous, ½ cup		17	
Coriander, fresh ¼ cup		*1*	
Cucumber, ½	*20*	*2*	*0.4*
Daikon (Lo Bok), ½ cup	*20*	*1*	*0.2*
Dandelion, raw, 2 cups		*5*	
Eggplant, ½ cup	*20*	*2*	*0.4*
Fava beans, ½ cup	79	17	13.4
Fennel, 1/6 bulb		*4*	
Gourd, ½ cup		12	
Garlic, 1 clov		*1*	
Green beans, ½ cup	*20*	*3*	*0.6*
Green peppers, ½ cup	*20*	*3*	*0.6*
Guacamole, 2 tbsp		*2*	
Hominy, ½ cup		23	
Hummus, 2 tbsp		*4*	
Kale, ½ cup		*2*	

Food	Glycemic Index	Net-Carb (g per serving)	Glycemic Load
Vegetables (continue...)			
Kidney beans, ½ cup	35	19.0	26.2
Kohlrabi, ½ cup		4.4	
Leeks, 1	20	11.0	2.2
Lettuce, 1 cup	20	0.5	0.1
Lentils, ½ cup	30	16.0	4.8
Mung bean, 150 g	31	17.0	5.3
Mushrooms, fresh, ½ cup	20	1.0	0.2
Mustard green, 1 cup		1.0	
Navy beans, ½ cup	39	19.0	7.4
Okra, 4 oz	20	5.0	1.0
Onions, 1		8.0	2.0
Onions, green, ¼ cup	20	1.0	0.2
Parsnips, ½ cup	139	15.0	20.9
Pea soup, split with ham, 1 cup	66	56.0	37.0
Peas, green, ½ cup	48	11.0	5.3
Pinto beans, ½ cup	40	20.0	8.0
Popcorn, 1 cup	55	6.0	3.3
Potatoes, French fries, large	75	49.0	36.8
Potatoes, instant mashed, ½ cup	86	14.0	12.0
Potatoes, new, 5 small	62	23.0	14.3
Potatoes, red-skinned, baked, 1	93	15.0	14.0
Potatoes, white, 1	90	22.0	19.8
Pumpkin, fresh 1 cup	75	5.0	3.7
Quinoa, dry ¼ cup		28.0	
Radicchio, fresh 2 cups		4.0	
Radishes, 6	20	1.0	0.2
Rhubarb, ½ cup	20	2.0	0.4
Rutabaga, boiled ½ cup		8.0	
Semolina, 70 g	45	50.0	22.5
Seaweed, sushi 1 sheet		0.1	
Spinach, 1 cup	20	0.2	0.4
Squash, acorn, ½ cup	25	10.0	2.5
Squash, butternut, ½ cup	25	8.0	2.0
Squash, spaghetti, ½ cup	20	4.0	0.8
Squash, summer, ½ cup	20	1.0	0.2
Squash, zucchini, 1	20	3.0	0.6

Food	Glycemic Index	Net-Carb (g per serving)	Glycemic Load
Vegetables (continue...)			
Sweet potatoes, mashed, ½ cup	54	20.0	10.8
Soy beans, ½ cup	*18*	*10.0*	*1.8*
Soy milk, unsweetened, 1 cup	*31*	*1.0*	*3.1*
Swiss chard, ½ cup	*20*	*0.5*	*0.1*
Swiss chard, boiled, ½ cup		*2.0*	
Sweet potatoes, mashed, ½ cup	54	20.0	10.8
Taro, ½ cup	54	23.0	12.4
Tomato, 1 small	*23*	*3.0*	*0.7*
Tomato, cherry, 6	*23*	*4.0*	*0.9*
Tofu, firm, 4 oz	*20*	*2.0*	*0.4*
Tofu, silken, 4 oz	*23*	*3.0*	*0.7*
Turnips, ½ cup	*20*	*3.0*	*0.6*
Turnip greens, boiled, ½ cup		*1.0*	
Water chestnuts, ½ cup	*50*	*7.0*	*3.5*
Watercress, ½ cup	*20*	*0.0*	*0.1*
Yam, 3 oz	65	31.0	20.2
Yellow squash, ½ cup		*1.0*	
Sugar			
Fructose, 3 packets	23	10	2.3
Glucose, 2 ½ tablets	100	10	10.0
Honey, 1 tbs	58	16	9.3
Jelly beans, 10	80	26	20.8
Lactose, 7/10 oz	46	10	4.6
Maple syrup, 1 tbs	86	13	11.2
Molasses, 1 tbs	65	13	8.5
Sucrose, 1 tsp	65	4	2.6
Sugar, brown, 1 tsp	70	5	3.5
Sugar, white, 1 tsp	78	4	3.1
Syrup, 1 cup	66	20	13.2

Food	Glycemic Index	Net-Carb (g per serving)	Glycemic Load
Bread and Cracker			
Angel food cake, 1 slice	67	17	11.4
Arrowroot cookies, 3	69	9	6.2
Bagel, 1 small	72	38	27.4
Banana bread, 1 slice	47	46	21.6
Biscuit, 1	79	27	21.3
Bread, Dark rye, 1 slice	76	18	13.7
Bread, hamburger bun, 1	61	22	13.4
Bread, kaiser roll, 1	73	34	24.8
Bread, Melba toast, 2	*70*	*7*	*4.9*
Bread, pita, whole wheat, 1	57	35	20.0
Bread, Pumpernickel, whole grain, 1 slice	51	15	7.7
Bread, Rye, 1 slice	65	15	9.8
Bread, Sourdough, 1 slice	52	20	10.4
Bread, white, 1 slice	70	12	8.4
Bread, whole wheat, 1 slice	69	13	9.0
Chapatti (wheat), 60 g	66	38	25.1
Cornbread, 1	49	21	10.3
Croissant, 1	67	27	18.1
Doughnut, 1	98	29	28.4
English muffin, 1	77	25	19.3
French toast, 1	58	18	10.4
Graham crackers, 4 squares	74	22	16.3
Italian bread, 1 piece	73	14	10.2
Matzos, plain, 1		28	
Muffin, 1	44	28	12.3
Oatmeal cookies, 2	55	12	6.6
Oatmeal, 1 cup	49	26	12.7
Pancake, 1	65	21	13.7
Pizza, cheese & tomato, 1 slice	60	28	16.8
Pound cake, 1 slice	54	42	22.7
Pretzels, 1	83	22	18.3
Rice cakes, 3	82	23	18.9
Ryvita, 25 g	63	18	11.3
Saltine crackers, 2	*74*	*4*	*3.0*
Short bread cookies, 4	64	19	12.2
Sponge cake, 1 slice	46	32	14.7
Vanilla wafers, 7	77	21	16.2
Waffles, 1	76	13	9.9
Wheat thin, 3	67	15	10.1

Food	Glycemic Index	Net-Carb (g per serving)	Glycemic Load
Cereal			
Bran Flakes, 1 cup	74	33	24.4
Corn Flakes, 1 cup	84	23	19.3
Cornmeal, 2 tbs	68	11	7.5
Cream of rice, ½ cup	70	14	9.8
Cream of wheat, ½ cup	71	14	9.9
Oatmeal, ½ cup	*49*	*10*	*4.9*
Oat Bran, 2 tbs	*55*	*6*	*3.3*
Raisin bran, 1 cup	73	39	28.5
Rice krispies, 1 cup	19	23	4.4
Rice, brown, ½ cup	55	21	11.6
Rice, white, ½ cup	66	22	14.5
Rice, wild, ½ cup	*50*	*16*	*8.0*
Wheat germ, 2 tbs	*60*	*5*	*3.0*
Dairy			
Buttermilk, 1% lowfat, 1 cup		13.0	
Half and half cream, 2 tbs	*30*	*1.0*	*0.3*
Cheese, Cheddar, 2 tbs		*0.2*	
Cheese, cream cheese, 2 tbs		*0.8*	
Cheese, creamed cottage, ½ cup	*3*		
Cheese, Feta, 2 tbs		*0.8*	
Cheese, Monterey Jack, 2 tbs		*0.1*	
Cheese, Ricotta, whole milk, ¼ cup		*1.9*	
Cream, 2 tbs	*25*	*1.0*	*0.3*
Ice cream, ½ cup	*61*	*16.0*	*9.8*
Ice milk, ½ cup	*50*	*15.0*	*7.5*
Milk, 2%, 1 cup	*30*	*12.0*	*3.6*
Milk, whole, 1 cup	*27*	*11.0*	*3.0*
Milk, skim, ½ cup	*32*	*6.0*	*3.8*
Milk, chocolate, 1 cup	34	16.0	5.4
Pudding, ½ cup	43	24.0	10.3
Sour cream, 2 tbs	*40*	*1.0*	*0.4*
Yogurt, fruit flavored, 8 oz	33	30.0	9.9
Yogurt, plain, 8 oz	*14*	*8.0*	*1.1*

Food	Glycemic Index	Net-Carb (g per serving)	Glycemic Load
Drinks and Junk Foods			
Apple pie, 1 slice	86	55	47.3
Beer, 1 can	60	13	7.8
Cherry pie, 1 slice	82	67	54.9
Chocolate, milk	34	16	5.4
Coca Cola, 1 can	63	39	24.6
Corn chips, 1 oz	72	16	11.5
Crab, imitation, 125 ml		7	
Custard, ½ cup	43	24	10.3
Gatorade, 1 cup	78	14	10.9
Power bar, 1	58	45	26.1
Potato chips, 10 pieces	76	10	7.6
Wine, white, 4 oz	*42*	*1*	*0.4*
Wine, red, 4 oz	*40*	*2*	*0.8*
Condiments			
Barbecue sauce, 2 tbs		*4.0*	
Cranberry sauce, 2 tbs		13.0	
Dijon mustard, 1 tsp		*0.5*	
Fish sauce, 1 tsp		*0.2*	
Gravy, ¼ cup		*3.0*	
Hollandaise sauce, 2 tbs		*0.3*	
Horseradish, 1 tsp		*0.4*	
Ketchup, 1 tbs		*4.0*	
Miso paste, 1 tbs		*3.0*	
Oyster sauce, 1 tbs		3.0	
Relish, 1 tbs		5.0	
Salsa, 1 tbs		*0.6*	
Spaghetti sauce, ¼ cup		*4.0*	
Soy sauce, 1 tbs		*1.0*	
Sweet and sour sauce, ¼ cup		15.0	
Tapioca, 250 g	*70*	*18.0*	*13*
Tartar sauce, 2 tbs		*1.0*	
Teriyaki sauce, 2 tbs		6.0	
Tomato sauce, ¼ cup		*4.0*	
Vinegar, balsamic, 1 tbs		*2.0*	
Vinegar, cider, 1 tbs		*1.0*	
Vinegar, red wine, 1 tbs		*0.0*	
Vinegar, sherry, 1 tbs		*1.0*	
Worcestershire sauce, 1 tsp		*1.0*	

Measurement Index

- tbs = tablespoon

- tsp = teaspoon

- 1 oz = 28.35 grams

- 16 fluid oz = 0.55 litre

- *Italic = Allow to use in Phase 3*

INDEX

A

B

C

C peptide - 30, 34, 35, 39, 45, 47, 50, 70, 71, 112, 243

C reactive protein - 62, 243

Calcium - 52, 85, 89, 91, 101, 116, 147, 163, 181, 183, 187, 188, 194, 196, 197, 198, 202, 203, 205, 206, 219, 220, 222, 235, 272, 287, 288, 303, 307, 319, 330, 334, 335, 349, 353

Canada Food Guide - 66, 68, 70, 113, 159, 174, 268, 301, 329

Cancer - 17, 24, 87, 88, 90, 139, 153, 217, 221, 228, 236, 259, 267, 316, 322, 323, 326, 329, 356

Carb counting - 48

Carnitine - 219

Central obesity - 36, 131, 212

Cholecystokinin - 136, 155, 264

Cholesterol - 11, 13, 17, 66, 73, 74, 75, 76, 77, 78, 79, 80, 81, 82, 84, 86, 92, 96, 111, 120, 121, 122, 123, 124, 125, 127, 128, 129, 134, 141, 153, 154, 156, 157, 159, 174, 175, 177, 178, 179, 180, 181, 183, 184, 185, 186, 187, 188, 189, 190, 191, 192, 193, 194, 195, 197, 198, 199, 200, 202, 203, 204, 205, 206, 208, 209, 218, 219, 220, 221, 223, 226, 228, 233, 234, 239, 240, 243, 246, 248, 253, 254, 255, 259, 263, 265, 269, 278, 279, 284, 288, 312, 316, 317, 319, 321, 331, 332, 337

Chromium picolinate - 93, 218, 222

Chronic fatigue syndrome - 24, 102, 220

CLA - 221

CoQ10 - 222

Coronary heart disease - 17, 24, 30, 36, 47, 65, 71, 78, 81, 83, 84, 114, 120, 124, 126, 127, 156, 157, 159, 167, 180, 209, 213, 218, 222, 227, 244, 284, 300, 356

Cushing's Syndrome - 63, 243

D

Da Qing Study - 41

Daily fluid intake - 267

Dawn phenomenon - 37, 38, 39

Diabetes, type 2 - 11, 19, 24, 25, 26, 27, 29, 30, 33, 36, 37, 39, 43, 44, 47, 50, 51, 52, 56, 57, 58, 60, 62, 64, 70, 72, 90, 92, 95, 112, 114, 120, 124, 135, 139, 161, 164, 224, 236, 244, 302, 360

Diet pills - 222, 332, 333

E

Essential amino acids - 36, 151, 258, 270, 319, 330, 334

Essential fatty acids - 136, 137, 153, 156, 246, 276, 278, 319, 320, 321, 330, 334

Exercise - 12, 13, 26, 38, 41, 42, 44, 47, 54, 60, 61, 69, 70, 75, 82, 85, 104, 112, 115, 116, 119, 123, 124, 126, 129, 130, 141, 143, 147, 148, 150, 207, 208, 209, 210, 211, 212, 213, 214, 215, 225, 226, 227, 228, 229, 231, 233, 235, 236, 241, 245, 276, 277, 287, 300, 301, 304, 316, 332, 335, 336, 345, 352, 356, 360

F

Fatty acids - 25, 26, 29, 43, 57, 58, 61, 72, 129, 136, 137, 145, 153, 155, 156, 175, 183, 221, 222, 230, 246, 266, 278, 317, 319, 320, 321, 330, 334

Fatty acids, essential - 136, 137, 153, 156, 246, 276, 278, 319, 320, 321, 330, 334

Fatty liver - 31, 95, 96, 112, 120, 124

Fibromyalgia - 11, 24, 102, 103, 104

Folic acid - 187, 194, 218, 222, 235

G

Glucagon - 27, 28, 37, 43, 61, 64, 139, 140, 141, 143, 149, 150, 254, 325, 330

Gluconeogenesis - 27, 28, 31, 36, 37, 38, 39, 41, 43, 45, 51, 53, 63, 64, 140, 149, 150, 230, 252, 262, 327, 330

Glucose intolerance - 29, 32, 63, 126, 162, 164

Glucose toxicity - 49

GLUT4 - 58

Glutamic acid decarboxylase antibody - 71, 151

Glycemic index - 167

Glycemic load -61, 69, 165, 169, 170, 171, 251, 253, 260, 266, 276, 302, 304, 330, 361, 362, 363, 364, 365, 366, 367, 368

Glycogen - 27, 28, 31, 38, 43, 45, 49, 58, 59, 76, 82, 91, 134, 140, 147, 207, 208, 211, 228, 230, 241, 242, 245, 252, 268, 271, 273, 305, 315, 316, 330

Gout - 17, 23, 76, 91, 101, 102, 139, 163

Growth hormone - 20, 100, 143, 144, 213

H

Hypertension - 11, 17, 24, 47, 51, 54, 71, 72, 84, 85, 86, 88, 92, 94, 99, 111, 112, 114, 119, 120, 123, 126, 129, 139, 208, 209, 220, 222, 226, 287, 311, 315, 333

Hypoglycemia, reactive - 142. 167

I

Ideal body fat range - 288

Insulin - 17, 18, 21, 25, 26, 27, 28, 29, 30, 31, 32, 33, 34, 35, 36, 37, 38, 39, 40, 41, 43, 44, 45, 46, 47, 48, 49, 50, 51, 53, 54, 55, 56, 57, 58, 59, 60, 61, 62, 63, 64, 65, 66, 69, 70, 71, 72, 73, 76, 81, 82, 83, 84, 85, 89, 90, 91, 92, 93, 94, 96, 100, 112, 113, 114, 117, 120, 124, 129, 130, 131, 134, 136, 139, 140, 141, 142, 143, 149, 150, 155, 161, 162, 163, 164, 165, 167, 169, 171, 182, 208, 209, 218, 220, 223, 228, 235, 236, 243, 253, 254, 263, 268, 270, 271, 276, 305, 316, 322, 323, 324, 325, 326, 327, 328, 330, 333, 360

Insulin receptors - 32, 61, 161

Insulin resistance - 17, 21, 25, 26, 30, 31, 32, 33, 34, 35, 36, 37, 38, 39, 41, 43, 44, 45, 47, 50, 53, 58, 62, 63, 64, 65, 66, 72, 73, 82, 83, 85, 90, 92, 93, 114, 120, 124, 129, 130, 131, 139, 141, 142, 161, 163, 164, 208, 218, 305

J

Jenny Craig's diet - 226, 332

K

Ketoacidosis - 53, 70, 71, 148, 149, 150

Ketones - 53, 56, 95, 126, 146, 147, 148, 149, 150, 151, 152, 162, 208, 219, 220, 266, 268, 277, 278, 289, 291, 315, 317, 319, 321, 330

Ketosis - 46, 53, 55, 95, 128, 145, 146, 147, 148, 149, 150, 151, 219, 228, 235, 262, 275, 276, 288, 290, 330

L

Legumes - 228, 235, 249, 250, 253, 258, 259, 260, 261, 265

Leptin - 62, 100, 113, 141

Lipoprotein lipase - 82, 332

M

N

O

P

Q

R

S

T

Target heart rate - 209

Thyroid - 20, 75, 76, 88, 136, 163, 164, 243

Triglycerides - 11, 20, 36, 37, 45, 55, 58, 66, 73, 74, 75, 76, 77, 81, 82, 86, 87, 92, 95, 111, 120, 121, 122, 123, 127, 134, 139, 145, 154, 155, 163, 167, 221, 222, 233, 239, 240, 243, 265, 290, 321, 330, 332

U

UKPDS - 49, 56, 57, 59, 60, 61, 62

Uric acid - 100, 101, 102, 124, 243

V

Vegan diet - 265

Vision, blurry - 40, 66

Vitamin - 26, 42, 86, 88, 183, 194, 217, 218, 219, 220, 221, 222, 229, 230, 232, 233, 235, 265, 271, 278, 290, 294, 300, 301, 304, 315, 319, 329, 330, 334, 348, 349

W

Waist circumference - 17, 18, 19, 28, 119, 121, 124, 125, 244

Water retention - 20, 23, 24, 64, 91, 92, 129, 139, 162, 163, 205, 249, 251, 283, 284, 287, 290, 315, 356

Weight Watcher's Diet - 227

Y

Z

Zone diet - 234

NOTES

NOTES

NOTES

NOTES